AF289831

Healing the Homeopathic Way

Uniting Shamanism, Alchemy and Modern Science

Jörg Wichmann

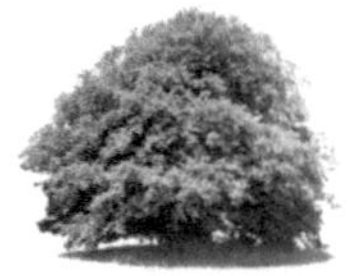

FAGUS – Publisher

Translation of the German book "Der Weg der Homöopathie"
(ISBN 978-3-933760-07-4), published by Fagus Verlag in 2019.

Proofreading and editing by Jenni Tree.

1st edition, January 2020
ISBN 978-3-933760-09-8
Printed in Germany by: Books on Demand
Cover design: Andrea Jakobs, Cologne, www.jakobs-design.de
Photo: Atropa belladonna, © Jörg Wichmann

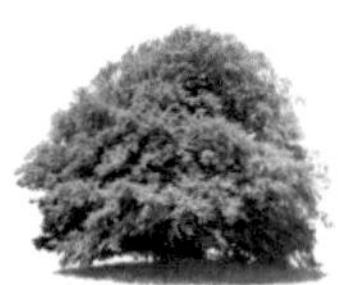

**FAGUS – Publisher
Jörg Wichmann
Eigen 81 –   D-51503 Rösrath
jw@provings.info**

2

Content

In the boxes highlighted in grey – in the table of contents in italics and indented – you will find additional information that relates to the topic in question but is not necessary for understanding and can be skipped in the text flow.

Introduction

Facing the crisis of modern health care, more and more people are looking for other, alternative and personally appropriate ways of healing. The first concern of many is to find a gentler healing method for themselves, whose possible side effects are no more dangerous than the disease to be cured. For others it is about not having to completely give up responsibility for themselves, their health and their lives in the healing process. Not only do they want to have their symptoms removed or their organs cured, they also want to be able to make sense of such a difficult phase of life as a disease and to mature personally from it.

Today, numerous holistic healing methods from different cultural contexts strive to do justice to this concern. Apart from the obvious differences, they all have a lot in common that is important for a comprehensive understanding of today's medical development. In a new way, this book presents a path that is based on and promotes our own inner healing powers: classical homeopathy, the most important alternative to the predominant mechanistic medicine for more than two hundred years.[1]

Holistic healing methods are not only healing methods for use when you are ill, but are also part of a world view that helps us live healthily. A holistic view of the world gives us orientation and meaning and, through many of life's difficulties, helps us to stay healthy, creative and in balance. For many people this aspect is as important as the possibility of experiencing healing when ill.

Homeopathy is both known and unknown. Many people have come into contact with it through their own suffering or childhood diseases within the family. They have experienced homeopathy in practice and know that it is an effective method. However, many have found it difficult to find a good explanation as to *why* and *how* homeopathy *works*. There are many positive experiences, but behind them is often the question mark regarding what the successes are based upon. There are ideas of placebo, herbalism, talking cures, or vague understanding of 'vibrations' or 'energies' as effective factors – muddled and misguided understanding quite frequently.

Trying to explain the working of homeopathy in the same way as one generally understands the effect of a pharmaceutical medicine does not, however, lead to a real understanding. Moreover, the wrong view of the essence of homeopathic healing often prevents the full potential of this method from being realized. It is not enough to perceive homeopathy merely as a practical method. A healing method and the laws on which it is based can only be taken seriously if they fit into a world view that functions according to the same laws. Homeopathy often requires its patients and the public to accept that the effects of homeopathy lie outside the generally accepted reality, without being able to give an alternative world view in which it fits. The fact that homeopathic treatment works and heals convinces many people. But there remains an uneasiness to get involved in a system that contradicts lots of everyday assumptions about our world, or at least seems not to provide clear information about these connections. In trying to deconstruct and understand our world in its minutest material parts, the spirit of the whole is lost, subsumed into the sum of its parts. The mechanistic world view has no place for the sacred, the divine, the magical, that which is not 'countable' – the unaccountable.

For this reason, many more or less scientific pseudo explanations are put together, which are then rejected again and again by the established science. All attempts to understand homeopathy through by way of the current conventional science are bound to fail because such science is not the appropriate world view. Rather, homeopathy is based on a world view that is initially very unusual for many people. Homeopathy[2] is part of an ancient European spiritual tradition that differs fundamentally from the mechanistic thinking of the currently established materialistic sciences. Only from the wealth of thoughts and experiences of hermetics and alchemy, even reaching into the world of shamanism, do the principles and procedures of homeopathy make recognisable sense. Once we have understood the essence of these

6

ancient traditions, this treasure of knowledge that unites all humanity, will the mysteries of homeopathy be solved in a simple way. And we can trust that a constantly evolving materialistic science is in the process of approaching the insights of this *philosophia perennis*, the eternal philosophy, on its own paths. We will discuss this in a later chapter.

Much of what is said here for homeopathy also applies analogously to other holistic healing methods. The holistic healing methods are neither remnants from a 'pre-scientific' era, whose semi-understood experiences have to be scientifically processed, nor are they forms of a 'complementary' medicine, which can complement the actual and main medicine, where less problematic ailments are concerned. Rather, they are complete and independent fields of knowledge and methods, with their respective strengths and weaknesses, which can in principle be used for the healing of all human diseases.

They are therefore not only alternative methods for the treatment of diseases, but they also share the ground of a world view that could be transformative in today's crises. This combination of properties offers challenge and opportunities: it is a system of healing whose infinite possibilities are known to but a few, and even then only in part.

By associating the healing method of classical homeopathy with shamanic healing and seeing the preparation of its remedies as an alchemical procedure, it is possible to fully and profoundly understand this method of healing, which has so far been unsatisfactorily explained. In this understanding it can be taken by therapists as well as by patients as a fascinating way to find access to one's own healing powers, to find healing in the deep encounter between people and between people and the world and thus to gain an expanded relationship to oneself, one's fellow human beings and the environment.

With this, homeopathy says goodbye to the struggle for so-called scientific recognition and classification into a world view that does not fit in with holistic healing methods. In fact, it has always been possible to prove the existence of homeopathic effects within the conditions of basic science; but there are also scientific theoretical reasons for the fact that an explanation of this effectiveness will not be satisfactorily possible within the given framework. However, it's a mental shortcut that something that cannot be explained mechanistically, generally cannot be explained.

Homeopathy is easy to explain and understand, but not within the framework of today's mechanistic science. With this book I would like to try and shed light on the spiritual background of this way of healing and to explain the effect of homeopathic healing in this context.

Homeopathy was born a good two hundred years ago, when modern science was in its early stages of development; and a medicine similar to our present one was not yet in sight. With his new system, its founder Samuel Hahnemann, reverted to the old spiritual traditions of the Occident, but he was already a child of the Enlightenment and tried to formulate his discovery in the new terms. He even had the idea that with the help of homeopathy, medicine could become as exact and predictable as mathematics. These ideas of Hahnemann can be well understood from his time, because mathematical ideas, rationality and measurability were the intellectual programme of this epoch. But today they no longer help us to understand people, medicine or homeopathy. Today we know infinitely more about the possibilities and limits of modern science than Hahnemann could. And we can see today that homeopathy is much better understood on the basis of the world view that prevailed throughout Europe and the whole world before the rise of materialism and with which humanity has always tried to understand the world and its own existence, life and death, happiness and suffering.

This path to a clearer understanding of homeopathy and healing in general will lead us far back through alchemy to the shamanism of our very early ancestors, to the healing methods of native peoples and to esoteric approaches to understand the essence of being human. It will become clear that the production of homeopathic medicines is an alchemical process, and that the homeopathic approach to healing is most similar to shamanism. Thus homeopathy is rather alien to mechanistic science and orthodox medicine and can neither be understood nor judged by it. It does not contradict it, but has its own view of the world and its own scientific methods, which are comprehensive and conclusive in themselves.

8

Conversely, from the point of view of a holistic spiritual world view, one could ask what a suitable medicine could be? Among the forms of medicine developed in Europe, homeopathy as the most comprehensive system, osteopathy, which is becoming more and more important, anthroposophical medicine, Bach flowers and spiritual healing are the main forms of medicine to be considered. Although many of today's so-called 'alternative therapies' represent gentler alternatives to conventional medicine, they are essentially based on the same view of the world: herbal medicine, manual and chiropractic methods, forms of energy medicine such as bio resonance or electro acupuncture, most psychotherapies. Like orthodox medicine, they all assume a division between soul and body and believe that therapeutic measures have a causal influence on the system of body and soul.

Finally, in our consideration of the ways and possibilities of holistic healing, we will come across the extent to which this kind of healing is currently hindered in our society. In a liberal and pluralistic society, it should be self-evident that we citizens are not ideologically patronised or fixed in the choice of our way of life and our healing methods. In medicine, however, this is the case to a considerable extent. By becoming aware of the path we want to take in health and sickness and of the differences between the paths offered, we can gain the strength to work for greater freedom of choice.

There are different ways of knowledge and science that have their respective advantages and disadvantages, and different ways in which we can lead our lives. I would like to make a contribution to a partnership between different world views and lifestyles. Even though for me modern scientific thinking is the most exciting venture of the West and its greatest contribution to the development of the human spirit, I reject its claim to dominate all other views of the world. Genuine cooperation between different medical procedures and approaches will only be possible if there is an understanding and mutual respect for the particularities and differences involved. The aim of this book is to contribute to such a fruitful cooperation between different forms of science and medicine.

The book therefore has two aims: to show a path to homeopathy by embedding it in the larger context in which it belongs; and to enable interested people, patients and practitioners to find more clarity about different forms of therapy in order to consciously choose their own path in illness and health.

It is not the aim of this book to present or develop a particular or even new type of homeopathy. It is about understanding classical homeopathy better and understanding it as part of a larger mental environment. This better understanding will reveal some aspects of homeopathy that are still underdeveloped or have not been properly valued in their importance for the overall context of this holistic science. The mechanistic era of the West has forced homeopathy – as well as many other holistic sciences – to adopt a methodological approach that has atrophied a number of essential possibilities in these disciplines. Now that the end of this epoch is in sight in many respects, it is time to realise the full potential of holistic procedures and world-views and to begin their revival and implementation – for the benefit of countless 'sick' and 'healthy' individuals as well as the overall cultural development.

I had my first encounter with homeopathy during my training as a naturopath when I attended a lecture on the remedy *Symphytum* (*Symphytum officinale* is the Latin name for comfrey), which is typically used for acute complaints of the periosteum and joints. I had problems with my arm at the time, which I had broken 10 years earlier in the elbow joint and overloaded it a few months ago while working. Since then every movement in the elbow was painful and severely restricted, and I could feel a loose cartilage particle wandering around in the joint. For three months I had tried in vain to alleviate the complaints and tried all the methods I came across: sports ointments, bandages, compresses, essential oils, embrocations, warmth, cold; nothing had helped. Now I thought: Why not try a homeopathic remedy? So I took *Symphytum* in a low potency, but without seriously expecting that something would change noticeably. I didn't know anything about homeopathy yet, and the tiny globules didn't seem very impressive compared to my healing efforts so far. In fact, however, the next morning the pain was so intense that I only had a few centimetres reach to move in the joint. The evening after, everything was gone, the pain and also this annoying and obstructive piece of cartilage in the joint. Like a spook, everything had disappeared and never came back.

I was very impressed, and I started to learn more intensively about homeopathy, which until then had not been my field of interest. I had to learn that such a miraculous healing process is very pleasant, but also rare. But such a chance hit, as I had experienced, showed me quite drastically the possibilities of a homeopathic remedy. Apparently my body was able to reintegrate even manifest cartilage parts in a very short time if it was given the right impulse. My interest was aroused and I was open for further new insights.

This marked the beginning of a phase in my life in which I experienced myself as a homeopathic patient, as a student of homeopathy and finally as a homeopathic practitioner and teacher. Today I am in all three roles at the same time: in homeopathy you remain a lifelong student – that is the beautiful and exciting thing about it –, I am a patient once and again, and homeopathic therapy has become my profession.

Ways of Homeopathic Healing

Health is the ability to develop symptoms in unhealthy situations and learn from them, I read recently.

This sentence reflects well the attitude of homeopathy towards health and disease. If you go to a homeopath for treatment, you will notice this first: He (or she) will be very interested in your symptoms, in your own experience. Medical diagnosis usually plays a subordinate role. Rather, as a homeopathic patient, you will learn to observe yourself very closely, which changes in your state of health occur under which circumstances, when they get better or worse, which likes and dislikes you feel, how your feelings and dreams react to your life. All this information gives homeopathic practitioners an overall picture on the basis of which they can prescribe a remedy. Everything is about understanding how you as a whole person, your mind and your organism, react to the situations of your life. Illness is a possible response to the demands of life and just as individual as any other behavioural pattern that someone can show. Everyone works, eats, sleeps, laughs, loves, scolds and runs in his or her typical way. But we believe we can summarise such a complicated event as a disease with a simple label. Hundreds of sick people with very different physical and mental states 'have rheumatism' and, depending on its severity, receive one or more typical medications. Their personal history and their own way of suffering are at best marginally perceived by an attentive doctor, but more likely ignored and considered unimportant for the 'rheumatism'.

The first and perhaps most important message of the homeopathic practitioner to the patients is: I take you and your condition, your own experience and your whole story seriously, every detail of it as you have experienced and suffered it yourself. I listen to everything quietly, without judging or interpreting anything. With this form of therapy you yourself as a whole person are in demand and challenged. It is about you, about your life and your unique way to be ill, to suffer, to become healthy and to shape your existence. The therapy can promote and support you in your own power and invite you to use your illness as an opportunity for greater self-awareness and to continue on your path strengthened and healed. Homeopathic treatment gives the impulse and shows the way. You yourself go out on your own.

This basic attitude has various components that are also helpful in life. Listening calmly without evaluating or reinterpreting is a key to deeper understanding and greater openness and closeness in all human contacts and also in nature. Ultimately, my whole biography is a kind of anamnesis of life with myself – '*an-amnesis*', retrieving from the unconscious, from oblivion. If I take this attentive and non-judgmental look at my life span, I can gradually discover what my soul meant by my existence. Looking at myself in the same way as a good therapist would do, can be a helpful exercise in freeing myself from the judgements of a strict superego, taking myself more lovingly and leniently, or even finding out my own excuses.

The approach of always wanting to perceive the whole thing and not just correcting the symptoms alone is not only useful in healing, but also helps me everywhere in life where I want to understand connections, where a project does not run as I imagined it to or where I want to gain a better overview of political events. Looking at the specifics from the perspective of the whole makes everything more transparent.

And the idea that my body knows the best solution and only needs a small impulse to move towards healing gives great confidence that the power for my life lies within myself and not in external help, experts or gurus.

Remedies and Similarity – the Simile Principle

Usually all attention in homeopathic therapy is focused on the prescription of a homeopathic remedy – both on the part of the patient and in homeopathic education. It forms an essential part, but only a part, of the comprehensive concept of homeopathy considering ourselves and life. Yet since homeopathic medicine in general is the starting point of many discussions about this form of therapy, we want to begin our walk along the homeopathic paths with it.

According to the individual approach, as indicated above, within homeopathy a remedy is not prescribed with regard to a specific diagnosis of a disease, but in the greatest possible similarity to the nature of the patient and to the essence of his or her disease. '*Similia similibus curentur*' – Similar things should be cured by similar things, that is the so-called Principle of Similarity or Simile principle. This similarity means that a substance in homeopathic treatment is able to heal such a complex of symptoms as it causes in a healthy person in the context of a remedy proving (or poisoning).

The practical work of homeopaths with their remedies now consists, on the one hand, in finding out the properties of possible remedies through remedy provings (usually on groups of colleagues) and, on the other hand, in determining by means of detailed case taking – the anamnesis – which of the known medicines is the most similar to the condition to be cured in the respective patient.

Samuel Hahnemann, the founder of homeopathy, came across this law of similars when he was translating a medical book and wanted to check a claim about the effects of cinchona bark (*China officinalis*). He simply took it for a few days and to his surprise noticed that this substance caused very typical malaria symptoms in him as a healthy person. At that time, cinchona bark was the main medical remedy for this serious tropical disease, and even today, conventional medicine still uses chemically modified extracts from cinchona bark against malaria. Hahnemann thus experienced the symptoms against which the cinchona bark was actually used – triggered by the remedy itself. He continued to experiment, on himself and on family members, and found out that he had come across a general principle which had also been formulated by ancient doctors, such as the famous Hippocrates, and the most important physician of the late Middle Ages, Paracelsus.

As an educated and well-read scholar, Hahnemann will certainly have known of the ideas of his predecessors about healing by way of similars, but it was in the spirit of his time that he relied on an assumption only when he could confirm it by trials. Hahnemann spent the rest of his life researching this idea further, proving new remedies and systematising the results, refining the rules of his healing method and working out a form of preparation of the 'homeopathic' remedies (as he then called them) that met his high demands for a fast, gentle and lasting medicine.

Identifying the substance that comes closest to the overall picture of the patient's symptoms, finding the most similar remedy, is not an easy task. After all, from hundreds of known remedies with partly quite similar characteristics, the most similar is to be found. The result also depends on how well the therapist has understood the patient's problems, because during the first conversations often only the surface of the actual story is revealed.

A very simple example for illustration: A patient comes to my practice because she complains about sore throats that have been getting worse for three days. I can already sense her grumpy, defensive nature. I let her tell about it: The sore throat stings, especially when swallowing, and gets worse when she moves her head. She also complains of a terrible thirst. She does not see a reason for the sore throat; she has not caught a cold and has no other symptoms.
On questioning, the patient explains that she does not like to move now in general and that the way to my practice had already been too much for her. This corresponds to my initial perception of her mood. The homeopathic medicine that will help her is Bryonia, the wild hop plant. The typical signs of this remedy are so well known that I don't have to read about it.
To be on the safe side, I ask her if she would rather be alone or in company during this disease; and she confirms my assumption that she prefers to be left alone and otherwise reacts rather grumpily. But I'm not satisfied with that yet, because I sense another kind of emotion in the background, and so I'm sure that's not the whole story yet. Knowing this patient, I believe that it would be important and helpful for her to be able to further extend the overall picture of her sore throat. Therefore I ask her to tell me about her experiences and moods of the last days. She then reports that they are about to move into a new house, the financing of which has been secured, but she would still give it a lot of thought. Just three days ago, her husband and she had had an

appointment at the bank. As she tells this, she notices for herself that the sore throat has occurred exactly since that date. She laughs about this spontaneous insight, gets her remedy and goes home.
Fears for the property and the business are known from the remedy picture 'Bryonia'. Speaking metaphorically: The garden fence is very important for wild hops, because they have to climb up it.

The decisive factor for the choice of the remedy was not the occurrence of a sore throat per se, but the typical stabbing pain character, which could also have manifested itself in the bladder or cough, as well as the strong thirst and aggravation of the discomfort with every movement.

With regard to the case history, it should also be noted that financial worries are not considered to be 'psychological' causes of sore throats. In the homeopathic sense they are part of the totality of a complaint, a pattern that appears analogously on different levels. However, the psychological side of the symptoms is usually closer to our experience, our ego, and easier to 'understand' than the physical symptoms. That is why it is easier to restore conscious contact with our whole life through them. The encounter with the homeopathic medicine *Bryonia* will first help the patient to get rid of her sore throat (in this case until the next morning) and in the long run reduce her fears for material safety. Such changes can sometimes be experienced through dreams and often through more or less unconscious inner changes in everyday life. Therapeutic accompaniment of this process can also provide a deeper understanding of the need for security and stability.

Even Hahnemann, at a time when psychology was still a long way from being a science, recognised that mental states – he called them mind symptoms – are most important for the individual understanding of a state of illness. However – and this is the special advantage of the homeopathic method – all physical states and sensations are taken seriously as expressions of the body and integrated into the overall picture. This overall picture is the homeopathic 'diagnosis', the characteristic pattern which includes all levels of the human being and within homeopathy bears the name of the natural substance which, according to our experience, is most similar to it. The patient presented above is therefore suffering from a *'Bryonia'* disease. In homeopathy, diagnosis and therapy coincide. Once I have recognised the condition, I also know the remedy – ideally. Theoretically, there is an infinite number of different remedies, herbal, animal, mineral, chemical and other substances that can be used in homeopathic preparations and would produce typical conditions in provings. No one could ever overlook such abundance. Hahnemann worked with about ninety different remedies; today many hundred remedies are quite well known and proved, and new ones are constantly being added. Therefore in a real case the similarity to a condition can usually only be met with moderate exactness. Often one must approach a condition with several remedies; or as a therapist I am facing a condition, which I can describe exactly and typically, yet I don't know any homeopathic remedy, which corresponds to it well. Then I can only hope that in discussions with colleagues, by further reading or by the homeopathic proving of new substances, I come across the suitable remedy for this person. Fortunately such cases are rather rare, and we can help satisfactorily with the remedies known to us in general. In the chapter after next we will deal in detail with the subtle interaction of practitioner, patient and remedy.

The fascination of the diagnoses '*Bryonia*', '*Lachesis*' or '*Natrum muriaticum*' compared to clinical diagnoses is that the patient receives a mirror of his or her inner and outer state with the remedy, i.e. a substance of the world as a possible help for self-knowledge. It is not necessary for the homeopathic healing that the patients know or observe this, but it can be very exciting for an extended understanding of the healing process and for the extension of one's own consciousness to deal with it.

Ignatia amara
The Ignatius bean is used in states where the basic tendency is cramping and which leads to paradoxical reactions and great hypersensitivity. The best known feature is the adherence to grief or disappointment in which a person cannot resign him- or herself to a loss. The blocked feelings manifest themselves in silent brooding, violent sighs or hysterical outbursts. All states can change quickly or turn into their opposite, crying in laughter, brooding in fury. All feelings are experienced very intensely, but the romantic inner life easily comes into conflict with external demands for rationality. Experiencing the strong inner contradictions can lead to hysteria or fainting. Typical for the feeling of internal cramp is a lump sensation in the throat, sighing, nervous shivering and muscle cramps, up to and including chorea, and also shows up as twitching of facial and other muscles, eyelid cramps, stomach cramps, hiccups, cough cramps, swallowing cramps, urge to urinate simultaneous with the inability to urinate, spasmodic yawning. Sleep is superficial, and the limbs twitch a lot. In general, strong feelings worsen all complaints, as do stimulants such as coffee and tobacco. Pressure, loneliness, deep breathing, travelling and changes in position, on the other hand, improve. Another set of paradoxical symptoms are: Appetite, which disappears when the food is there; nausea, which gets better by eating indigestible things; roaring in the ear, which gets better by music; coughing stimulus, which gets worse by coughing. Ignatia has an aversion to meat, alcohol and especially smoking.

Nux vomica
Similarly overexcited is the patient, who is helped by *Nux vomica*, the poison nut tree, but here the organism shows signs of strong over-excitation, which easily occur in the modern urban lifestyle. Excessive work and ambition, stimulants and drugs, insomnia and overnight stays, too much and irregular food, material worries and lack of exercise lead

to the typical picture of *Nux vomica* disease with its focus on nervous reaction and digestion. *Nux vomica* patients are very easily irritable, explode rapidly and put themselves and others under severe pressure – the typical choleric. They are very sensitive and hypersensitive to pain, noise and smells. Sleep is bad, comes late and is not restful. Moods alternate easily and violently, outbursts of anger are frequent. *Nux vomica* produces in healthy people the symptoms that we know from an excess of food, irritants and stress, and is therefore often used homeopathically to alleviate the consequences of overdose of any kind. Nausea, choking and vomiting as well as colic, abdominal pain and constipation often occur. Vomiting, bowel movements and excretions of all kinds improve the symptoms. Sleep and warmth also help, because *Nux* patients are extremely chilly in physical exhaustion. Tension and spasticity also manifest themselves as asthma or acute back pain, for which *Nux vomica* provides excellent relief, provided the above-mentioned conditions are met.

Both *Ignatia* (bot.: *Strychnos ignatii*) and *Nux vomica* (bot.: *Strychnos nux vomica*) belong to the plant family *Loganiaceae* and contain to a large extent the poison Strychnine. Strychnine itself as a homeopathic remedy is similar to the medicinal pictures of *Ignatia* and *Nux vomica*, especially as far as the basic symptoms of cramps are concerned.

Dynamis and Potentisation

What about the second pillar of homeopathy, the homeopathic preparation of medicines? At first glance it seems quite simple: homeopathic medicines are produced by diluting a thoroughly ground (triturated) substance in a ratio of 1:100 and then rhythmically succussing it ten times, i.e. thumping it on a firm surface with the vial in your hand. This is the so-called *potentiation* or *potentisation* (see box for more details). Potentiated agents are marked with C and a number indicating the number of potentisation steps performed (dilution plus shaking). In the case of a '*Lachesis* C12', the initial substance, the poison of the bushmaster snake, would have been diluted twelve times in a ratio of 1:100 and rhythmically shaken. It is easy to calculate that with potencies above C12, no molecule of the starting substance is present. This is the reason why scientific minds tend to be bewildered, stating Avogadro's constant as their chemical reason, but homeopathy is not a form of chemical therapy. The effect is not based on the chemical ingredients. Otherwise it would be completely nonsensical to produce potencies up to millions. Even the most common potency levels of C30 and C200 used in classical homeopathy indicate dilutions in which chemically nothing has been detectable for a long time. No homeopath would be so stupid as to overlook that fact. Therefore, the discussions about the fact that there is 'nothing in it' completely miss the point. One would have to claim that every conceivable effect must always be chemical. That's nonsense, of course. From a chemical point of view, two CDs or two books cannot be distinguished either and certainly not checked for the sense of their content.

The character of a homeopathic potency is rather that of information. The homeopathic remedy conveys a message to our holistic system (or organism) or body, life force, mind and spirit – an impulse, how to achieve a better balance. Hahnemann's idea of this was that a homeopathic remedy causes an artificial disease in the sick as well as in healthy people during remedy testing (called 'proving' in homeopathy). In the case of the patient, however, it is so similar to the already existing disease that it eradicates it. We can also use the modern technical image of *resonance* to form an idea of it: similar to a tuned resonance event. Or we can imagine the homeopathic remedy to strengthen the information existing in the organism in the same sense (i.e. *homeo*-pathically) in such a way that the life force can finally react correctly to it. All these images and aids to understanding have in common the fact that they do not have a material or energetic effect, but rather a transmission of information. This also makes it understandable that the remedy be administered in very small and very rare doses – the better and more precisely it works, the less frequently it is to be applied. It's like with good advice: If I give it at the right time and in the right way, I don't have to repeat it. If I have to scream it out loud more than once, there's something wrong with my piece of advice. What happens due to a proper homeopathic impulse is the self-reaction of the organism, or the dynamis, its life force.

In the potentisation of remedies Hahnemann saw a possibility to strengthen the dynamic or spiritual nature of a substance[3] and at the same time to reduce or exclude the physically toxic effects by dilution. As the cause of an illness he saw the 'morbid derangement', a disharmony of the life force of a person, of the 'dynamis' as he called it. Therefore, a remedy should not act directly on the physical body, but on the dynamis, whose derangement shows itself externally as a 'disease'. This derangement or disharmony can have various causes, which of course must also be eliminated. But the most important thing for healing is *how* this derangement is, i.e. *how* an organism (meaning the interaction of body, life force, soul and spirit) reacts to a situation, to an external stimulus. Hahnemann said that we cannot really know anything about the inner nature of the disease. We must adhere to the signs, to the symptoms that a person shows us. These are the expressions of the way in which the dynamis is out of tune and how it can therefore be healed. In Hahnemann's view, the physical level of existence is only a carrier of signs; life, health and illness take place on another level, which we cannot directly perceive. Hahnemann's contemporary Goethe put it this way: "Everything transitory is only a parable." So it is by no means a consequence of Hahnemann's ignorance of molecular processes and the later-discovered Avogadro number that he brought his potencies into levels of dilution where no materiality remained. Rather, this is the very principle of his healing

22

method. Like alchemists, he was concerned with liberating the essence or spirit of a substance from its coarse materiality. The idea as such is ancient, but the potentisation process is probably a genuine invention of Hahnemann's. One can even say that a potentised remedy works the longer, deeper and more intensively, the higher the potency; the further away from the materiality.

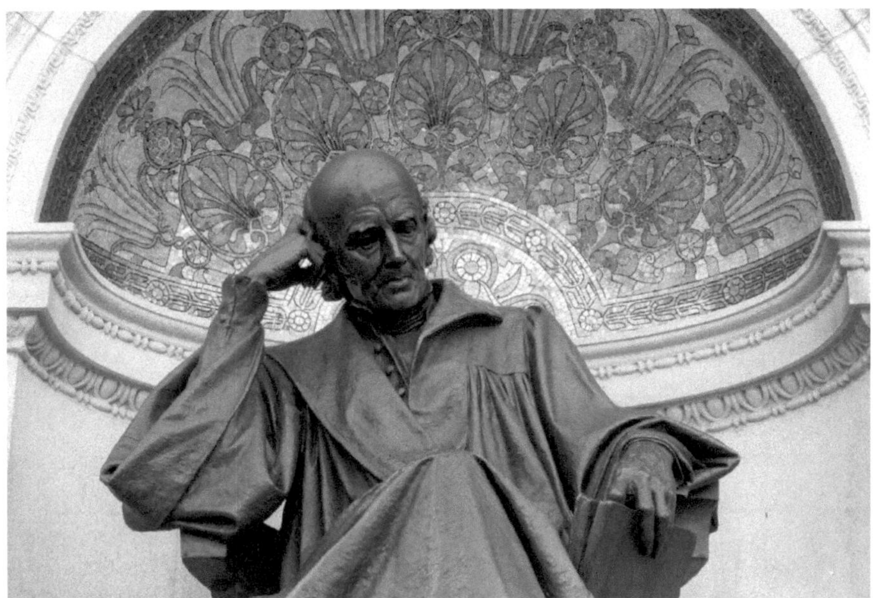

Hahnemann statue at Scott Circle, Washington DC

Samuel Hahnemann – a Short Biography

Christian Friedrich Samuel Hahnemann was born on April 10th 1755 in Meissen, the son of a porcelain painter in simple circumstances, and died on July 2nd 1843 in Paris as a famous physician.

The first half of his life was marked by unrest and homelessness. With many children and little money, the Hahnemann family travelled for many years through the German countryside with a covered wagon, always looking for a permanent home and nourishing work. Hahnemann had given up his medical practice because he was unable to justify the use of the contemporary medical methods on his patients, and so earned his living by translating chemical and pharmaceutical reference books, as well as conducting small research projects and publications of his own.

From 1821 to 1835 he ran an orderly homeopathic practice in the Saxon town of Köthen (Coethen), developed his teaching further, and conducted numerous remedy provings. A few years after the death of his wife Henriette, he married at the age of eighty the much younger noble Frenchwoman Melanie d´Hervilly, with whom he settled in Paris and shared a practice that became internationally famous.

Hahnemann's most important written works were:

1793-99 – the pharmacist's encyclopaedia in four volumes, the *Heilkunde der Erfahrung* (*Medicine of Experience*).

1805 – *Organon of the Rational Art of Healing*.

1810 – later edition *Organon of the Healing Art*.

1811-21 – *Materia Medica Pura* (*Reine Arzneimittellehre*).

1828-30 – *Chronic Diseases*

1842 – and a manuscript of the 6th edition of the *Organon*

In 1790 he discovered the principle of the simile in his experiment with Cinchona bark, which he published in 1796.

He first mentioned the term *homeopathy* in 1807, and *potentisation* (or *potentiation*) in 1827.

As you could see from the last description, the entire procedure makes no sense at all within a mechanistic scientific framework. Rather, the material level is consciously abandoned both in the understanding of diseases and in the practical production of remedies. Above this, the idea of similarity also plays no role in the mechanistic thinking of modern science. Their thinking is linear: cause and effect follow physical and chemical principles of action. That substances or beings of nature have a correspondence with each other or can interact with each other because they are 'similar' does not make any sense in established scientific thinking. Although Hahnemann strove to be as precise as possible and relied meticulously on his observations, he did not inhabit the world view that we know today as the modern sciences. In the next chapter we will follow this other world view and science more closely and now turn back to homeopathy.

"Medicinal substances are not dead substances in the ordinary sense; rather their true essence is merely dynamic, spiritual – is pure power ..."
(Hahnemann, *Materia Medica Pura*, Part 6, p. 11)

"It is not the physical atoms of these highly dynamised medicines nor their physical or mathematical surface (with which one wants to interpret the higher forces of the dynamised medicines, still materially enough, but in vain), that the medicinal energy is found. More likely, in the moistened globules or in their solution, there lies invisible an unveiled, liberated, specific, medicinal power contained in the medicinal substance, which acts dynamically in contact with the living animal fibre upon the whole organism (without communicating anything material however highly attenuated). It acts more strongly the more free and immaterial this energy has become through the dynamisation."
(Hahnemann, *Organon*, §11, Note)

"It is very likely that matter, by means of such dynamisation (development of its true, inner, medicinal essence), will dissolve completely into its individual spirit-like being in the end and can therefore, in its crude state, only be regarded as consisting of this undeveloped, spiritual essence."
(Hahnemann, *Organon*, §270, Note 7)

Hahnemann describes the potentisation in *Organon* §270 (abbreviated):
"In order to best effect this development of power, a small part of the substance to be dynamised, such as one grain [an old unit of measuring mass, 62 mg, equalling more or less a grain of cereal], is first diluted by triturating it with three times 100 grains of lactose for three hours in the manner specified below, until it is diluted a million times. For reasons given below, a grain of this powder is first dissolved in 500 drops of a mixture consisting of one part brandy and four parts distilled water, a single drop of which is placed in a vial. To this you add 100 drops of pure alcohol and then give the bottle, which has been grafted with its stopper, 100 strong succussions with the hand against a hard, but elastic body. This is the medicine in the first degree of dynamisation, with which fine sugar globules are first moistened, then quickly spread out on blotting paper, dried and stored in a well-corked vial with the sign of the first (I) degree of potency. From this, only a single globule is taken for further dynamisation, put into a second, new vial (with a drop of water to dissolve it)

and then dynamised with 100 drops of good rectified spirit in the same way, by means of 100 strong succussions.

With this spirit-like medicinal fluid, again globules are moistened, spread out quickly on blotting paper, dried, kept in a well-corked vial from heat and daylight and provided with the sign of the second potency degree (II.). And so we continue until, through the same treatment, a dissolved globule XXIX with 100 drops of rectified alcohol, by means of 100 successions, has formed a spirit-like medicinal liquid, whereby the moistened and dried globules obtain the degree of dynamisation XXX.

Through this processing of crude medicinal substances, preparations are created, which only thus acquire the full ability to touch the suffering parts in the diseased organism aptly and thus to withdraw the sensation of the natural illness from the life principle present in them through similar, artificial disease affection. By this mechanical treatment, if it has been carried out properly according to the above teaching, it is caused that the medicinal substance, which in its raw state presents itself to us only as matter, sometimes even as unmedicinal material, by means of such higher and higher dynamisations, finally subtilises and transforms itself completely into spirit-like medicinal power, which in itself no longer falls into our senses, but for which the medicinally prepared globule, already dry, but much more so if dissolved in water, becomes the carrier and in this condition manifests the healing influence of that invisible power in the sick body."

Illness and Perception

With the approach described so far, homeopathy teaches us first: My illness is not something that only specialists can find in me. But my illness is what I can feel and perceive myself, on my body and also in my soul. I don't 'have tonsillitis' like hundreds of thousands of other Europeans in autumn too. It's just an imprecise label. Rather, I feel stabbing pain when swallowing, which is less outside than in a warm room; I can swallow dry things more easily than liquids, which seems very strange to me; furthermore, the pain in the morning when I wake up is much worse; I sweat much more than usual, especially at night.

We have largely lost this kind of exact perception of ourselves – we have never been asked about it, it was considered unimportant, 'subjective' or even imaginary. We have learnt to pass over our perceptions and instead think in terms of labels. In the course of a homeopathic treatment we learn again to observe ourselves very closely. We get to know processes and rhythms of our body and our energy balance that have always been there. It opens up a part of our inner world that we didn't know that way. This brings the illness closer to us and we experience that we do not 'have' an illness like an uninvited guest whom we can send away again. Rather, we *are* ill, the illness is a form of expression that fits into a pattern of our personality structure, albeit in a very unpleasant or even threatening way. Because this fact is so important and yet so unfamiliar, I would like to repeat it once again: **My way of being ill is an expression of my life as unique as my fingerprint, just as typical of my being as my handwriting, my way of working, painting, speaking and loving. Illness does not afflict me, but is part of my individual way of reacting to the demands of life, processing them or repulsing them. And only on this – very individual – level is it possible to find a different solution for my life's tasks and problems than getting ill.** (Incidentally, it should be noted that there are also supra-individual diseases, epidemics, that follow other laws and have to be considered differently. But that should be left out for the time being.)

Direct observations today are either completely ignored or they are very quickly interpreted and psychologically classified. In this respect it is very valuable to practice and refine the exact perception before all interpretation and theory. This self-perception produces an overall picture, which is then matched from the homeopathic side with the picture of a remedy. In the encounter with the remedy we can then experience how some features of our pattern change, how painful or dysfunctional aspects of the pattern change into more constructive ones, or how patterns from the past sometimes reappear. Thus, health and self-awareness increase equally. Conversely, the practitioner also depends on the patients' increasingly differentiated self-awareness and self-observation. Complex disease states often cannot be fully recognised and understood at first glance. Homeopathic treatment is a joint journey of patient and practitioner, in which precise observation and precise selection of a remedy complement each other. This means that patients never feel that they are just the object of treatment. Rather, they learn to trust in their own strength and intuition. And ultimately healing occurs where the knot loosens completely, where we can clearly recognise, accept and balance our patterns.

Hahnemann as well as many of his successors did not consider this aspect of consciousness to be important. Of course, homeopathy can heal living beings that do not have the ability to self-reflect, or even to heal people without any involvement of their consciousness. However, Hahnemann clearly stated in his late years that his previous approach to homeopathy did not lead to a complete cure (see next box). Until his death he was working to develop his miasm theory of chronic diseases, because he knew that his homeopathic approach needed a further understanding to make healing permanent and to prevent the constant shifting of symptoms that is typical of so many forms of therapy. From the point of view of today's manifold therapy experiences and also in recourse to those healing methods on the basis of which homeopathy came into being (without Hahnemann being aware of this), I dare to assume that precisely this component of self-reflecting consciousness could be a decisive factor, at least for the modern adult human being, having been missed by Hahnemann, in order to achieve a really stable state of health. If practitioner and patient go down this path together, homeopathy can be an ideal instrument for this.

"Usually, however, after often attempting to defeat the ill, which is always changing and reappearing again, there were complaints left which by the many homeopathic remedies which had been proved so far, had to be left unerased and often even undiminished – always other and again other complaints, also probably more and more troublesome and in the following time more serious – even with the patient's impeccable way of life and punctual obedience. Basically the chronic infirmity could be stopped by all this only little in its progress by the homeopathic physician and worsened nevertheless from year to year.

This was and remained the faster or slower process of such cures of all unvenerable, considerable, chronic diseases, even if they seemed to be conducted exactly according to the teachings of the homeopathic art known up to this point. Their beginning was pleasant, the continuation less favorable, the outcome hopeless."

(Hahnemann, *Chronic Diseases*, Vol. I, Preface)

The Healing Process

Once again back to the homeopathic practice. So far, we have become acquainted with the two main pillars of homeopathic work:
the law of similarity and
the potentisation of remedies.
In addition, we have encountered remedy proving as the most important method of gaining knowledge about remedies. It became apparent that homeopathy is a holistic form of therapy with its own laws. It looks back on more than two hundred years of systematic experience and is by no means a complementary kind of medicine to the currently predominant orthodox medicine. Rather, it is a medicine that is aimed at the whole person and can deal with any type of disease.

The holistic dimension also includes the temporal dimension: During a homeopathic treatment, earlier symptoms often recur, often running backwards in the order of their occurrence. It looks as if the organism, with the help of its healthy life force, is also taking the 'skeletons out of the closet' and working up old problems that had to be suppressed beforehand. The restoration of the whole of life also happens lawfully on the temporal line. We are only comprehensively healthy if we have also brought light into our past. The process of holistic healing does not distinguish between mental and physical trauma. All levels of experience are rolled up until the process has touched all layers of a human being and all stages of his life. Those who wish to quickly eliminate annoying complaints are not always well served with such a comprehensive healing approach. – Although a homeopathic therapy can also quickly and simply eliminate annoying complaints in simple cases, it only remains in the forefront of its full possibilities.

A holistic healing process often runs from the inside out or from the top down. This is due to the development of vital (often inner or upper) organs into less important ones. For example, asthma is more threatening to the organism than eczema, inflammation of the heart is more dangerous than joint inflammation, and so on. Skin phenomena often migrate from the head over the torso to the legs in order to finally disappear completely. A development of symptoms in this direction is therefore considered to be favourable in the context of homeopathic or any other holistic treatment; conversely, if a skin rash disappears but asthmatic symptoms occur, this is regarded as a sign of 'suppression' of the disease, i.e. a worsening that is undesirable and requires a new approach to the healing process. In conventional medicine, which does not take these holistic laws into account, such oppressive processes occur again and again, without these connections even attracting attention. For the newly occurring symptoms either another specialist is responsible, or the connection is not considered possible for theoretical reasons and therefore usually not even observed.

In case important reaction areas of the organism are blocked by means of cortisone, antihistamines, hormones or several other substances, the possibilities of the development of vital force are restricted to such an extent that a homeopathic remedy can hardly show any effect. This is the reason why homeopathy can only be used as a 'complement' or 'addition' to orthodox medicine in exceptional cases. Both forms of treatment contradict each other and pursue the opposite goal. Homeopathic treatment promotes the organism's own reactions, while orthodox medicine often suppresses them and prevents them on a chemical level.

During Hahnemann's lifetime and even a hundred years later, the oppressive possibilities of medicine were different from today – there were no vaccinations, no antibiotics or cortisone. And only very few people could afford the academic medicine of the time (which saved them a lot of suffering). Therefore, the early homeopaths often still saw very clear and regular healing processes. Today almost all patients who come for homeopathic treatment have already taken a pile of medicines, are vaccinated many times and are under the constant influence of an unmanageable mass of environmental and 'pleasure' chemicals. The result is not only a confused tangle of suppressed and repeatedly suppressed symptom complexes but also a series of 'medical diseases' or 'artificial diseases', as Hahnemann called them. By this he meant diseases that were not caused by the adversities of life, but were caused by man himself through the use of poisons or harmful 'treatment' methods. Hahnemann considered such complaints to be homeopathically untreatable. Fortunately, he was not quite right with this assessment, otherwise a homeopathic practice would no longer be

30

possible today. But it is true that most of the disease and healing processes that we observe today only follow the rules formulated by the fathers of homeopathy in phases. Many processes are confusing, jump back and forth between symptom complexes and can only be healed by patient and constant further treatment.

Today the balance can only be restored more laboriously than two hundred years ago because of our different way of life. But then, as now, it's about the same goal. The prescribed homeopathic remedy is a precise stimulus which causes the vital energy, the dynamis, to fulfil its task more fully and to restore and maintain the wholeness of the organism according to its laws. It is important to keep this in mind during difficult healing processes: the rules are not those of homeopathy or any other holistic procedure, but an organism must follow and is following the rules of life mediated by its dynamis. The healing is always based on the self-healing powers of the body, everything else is only incentives and support.

An often-observed rule of the homeopathic treatment is the so-called first reaction or 'initial aggravation'. This means that in many healing processes the state of the organism is stimulated in such a way that the symptoms are initially perceived as worsening in the first few hours (or days, depending on the disease), before they change to healing. The intensity and speed of the healing reaction depends entirely on the life force of the affected person. Acute diseases, which in homeopathy include all the ailments that occur in response to an external weakening of the life force, can heal quickly. Chronic illnesses are mostly more difficult to treat as they occupy the organism for years or decades and are often brought along as a so-called 'miasma' from family history. In therapy it is therefore important to distinguish between an acute occurrence of a disease in the homeopathic sense and a manifestation of a chronic disease. The terms acute and chronic have a different meaning in homeopathy than in orthodox medicine. An infection, for example, can be either an acute disease regardless of its symptoms, or it can be the flare-up of a chronic process that is now showing itself to be an infection.

Hahnemann explained the initial reaction to himself in such a way that a remedy always enforces a disease-like reaction of the organism.

The initial reaction then displaces the existing disease – provided that the 'similarity' between the two is large enough. And the secondary reaction of the organism to the stimulus set on it leads finally to healing. With this explanation he follows observations from his time about overlapping diseases, which can displace each other. Although this model does not stand up to a more thorough examination, it describes the course of natural healing processes quite well. Above all, however, Hahnemann has on this basis designed an approach to researching remedies that has been tried and proved many thousands of times to date. This is the homeopathic remedy proving of healthy individuals.

Remedy Provings

These provings are the most important source of homeopathic knowledge, on which the clinical observations are based. Hahnemann's practical basic work, *Materia Medica Pura*, is a collection of his first homeopathic remedy provings, a list of tens of thousands of symptoms. Hahnemann himself proved 99 remedies. After him thousands more provings have taken place, so that the homeopathic treasure of remedies today includes several hundred reasonably thoroughly proved remedies (not several thousand, as is often claimed). Several hundred other remedies are known only from practical applications, from poisoning symptoms or from herbal medicine, but are not thoroughly homeopathically treated. In principle, poisoning with a substance can be regarded as a simple remedy proving, which, however, due to the observation circumstances usually produces few differentiated results. Altogether almost nine thousand substances have appeared, been proved, used, mentioned or manufactured in the homeopathic context.4 Homeopathic remedy research therefore still has a broad field open to it, which has been intensively pursued internationally for several years – after a long break.

The possibility of remedy proving is based on the fact that the life force, the dynamis of healthy people, is also receptive to stimuli from high potencies and then produces characteristic symptoms on all levels of being (mental, spiritual, physical). We call the systematic generation and recording of such symptoms and signs a homeopathic remedy proving. According to Hahnemann, there is no fundamental difference between the generation of proving symptoms or healing by a substance. The life force always reacts to the stimulus in the same way, characteristic for this person and this substance. If there is already a similar disharmony in the vital force, the remedy stimulus superimposes the state of the disease and the counter-reaction of the dynamis erases the signs of the disease in the organism. If such a pathological condition is not present, the typical symptoms of the remedy simply appear in their pure form until the organism eliminates them again.

For example, I myself suffered from certain back and knee pains for almost two years after a beech (*Fagus sylvatica*) remedy proving. However, the initial reaction was pleasant and showed me a clear strength. I was able to assert myself well, was creative, in a good mood and had more fun at work. Every time I meet a beech in the forest, I am reminded that I was allowed to participate in its essence and special life energy. My relationship with the beech trees will always remain a special one, because I know that I am very receptive to their species, which means that I have reacted strongly to them in remedy proving. The unpleasant remains of this condition were later healed (after they had also taught me some things and served as an indicator for when I was out of balance) by my therapist with *Tilia*, the lime tree – interestingly also a native tree.

Thus homeopathy is obviously not 'naturopathy' in the sense that the body's defences should be strengthened in a natural way. Homeopathy does not work with the concept of the immune system and the remedies it uses are not 'natural' either. On the contrary, they are medicinal products which have been modified to a maximum degree and removed from their 'natural' state. In a certain sense, alchemistically speaking, it can be said that a substance is brought closer to its essence, that matter is brought to maturity by potentisation; but this is not 'natural' in the sense of naturopathic treatments, which try to positively influence the organism with water, light, food, fasting, movement, minerals, medicinal herbs, etc.. The praiseworthy and important endeavour of naturopathy to strengthen the strained body has nothing to do with the recognition of the mental picture or background of a disease, as homeopathy does. A healthy lifestyle can be helpful for homeopathy in that it helps to remove obstacles to healing, which Hahnemann already attached great importance to.

Even some homeopaths, especially in the popular literature, frequently say that the homeopathic method is harmless and, even if it is not useful, has at least no side effects. But anything that can heal can also make you sick. Even a harmless herbal tea, enjoyed at the wrong time and in excess, can cause symptoms. And our knowledge of homeopathic medicines is based precisely on their ability to cause symptoms in healthy people, the so-called proving symptoms. Without these sometimes quite drastic 'side effects', homeopathic remedy proving would be completely pointless. It is a basic law of homeopathy that a wrongly prescribed remedy can cause strong symptoms. This effect is desirable and necessary in remedy proving, but must be carefully considered in therapy.

A remedy proving takes place in the following way:[5] A group of interested people is brought together, mostly homeopaths themselves, ideally around 20 people. Among these, every one or two provers are assigned a supervisor, who observes and records the entire course of the proving, makes the initial anamnesis and is responsible for the health of the provers, i.e. breaks off the proving if the symptoms are too severe.

The provers take a potency between C6 and C200 of the substance (which is usually unknown to them) until clear symptoms appear. These are meticulously recorded in a diary to be kept a few days before the start of the proving until its end. In addition, there is daily contact between provers and supervisors to ensure additional external observation. If the symptoms subside again after a few days to two weeks, a looser follow-up takes place at larger intervals during two to three months. Afterwards all recorded symptoms, signs, moods, dreams and impressions are collected and evaluated, sorted, weighted and in a complex working process brought into the form by the proving management, which can then be published as a 'homeopathic remedy proving' of the respective remedy. The first collection of such results was Hahnemann's *Pure Materia Medica* (*Reine Arzneimittellehre*). It serves practising homeopaths as the basis for their prescriptions. Over the course of many years, it has become apparent which of the countless symptoms of a certain remedy frequently occur in patients and which could be cured by this remedy. Important things can thus be differentiated from unimportant things, typical things from the general ones; and little by little a clinically tested, reliable 'remedy picture' emerges, on the basis of which a homeopathic prescription can be made. The materia medica of homeopathic medicines contains a collection of proven and often confirmed symptoms for every common remedy, making them easier to manage. However, the text of the original proving of a remedy always remains the last instance to check how appropriate it really is in an individual case.

Already around the turn of the last century, detailed pharmacopoeias filled dozens of thick volumes, and today, without modern computer technology, the material accumulated over the course of two centuries by the international homeopathic community would be completely unmanageable. Today's homeopaths inform themselves about new remedy provings via the Internet.[6] Like all other knowledge in our cultural area, homeopathic knowledge has become incredibly complex and comprehensive. Whether we have become better practitioners as a result is another question.

"What is a doctor? He's the one who can cure the sick." (Paracelsus)[7]

"The doctor's highest and only profession is to heal sick people, which is called healing." (Hahnemann, *Organon* §1)

Health, Disease and Symptoms

At first glance, Hahnemann's sentence that it is important to "heal sick people" sounds almost trivial. In view of the development of modern medicine in particular, however, the question arises as to what we mean by a 'sick person' and when we can call ourselves 'healthy'. Modern medicine knows an incredible amount about diseases, but little about health. One of the most important laws of life is that I create what I concentrate on. A medicine that only takes care of diseases cannot make you healthy at all, at best symptom-free. And so health is often understood as freedom from symptoms: I feel healthy when I feel as little as possible of myself.

A symptom indicates that I am ill; but the symptom is not the illness. Making a symptom disappear has as little to do with overcoming illness as removing a warning light has to do with repairing a machine.

Already the use of language is treacherous: I 'have' an illness, like I have a car or little money, 'have' an illness like something coming from outside, which I want to get rid of. More correct would be to say, "I'm ill," or "I'm not well." The symptoms of illness indicate what is missing. Even the typical, often paternalistic medical question "Well, what's wrong with us?" has its wisdom, because what's wrong with one person is wrong with all of us. Individuality is an illusion, also in being ill. The individual sick person makes a problem of the whole community tangible; she or he is in this respect only a symptom.

So it would be more proper to say: I *am* ill, and this *being* ill is reflected in my symptoms. The symptoms are not only warning signals, but also signposts to 'what's wrong with me'. The fatal thing about orthodox medicine is not only the toxicity of its medication, but the fact that it clears away the signposts before you have understood its direction.

Does illness have a cause, or does it have an intention? This basic decision in the view of disease leads to very different approaches in its treatment. If illness primarily pursues an intention, then it would be pointless to eliminate its causes. Illness will then seek a new form of expression. The aim must then be to help it achieve its goal, if possible in a way that is more beneficial to the person than the course of the disease, if that is possible. The different forms of holistic therapy follow different paths to this end.

Gisela

For several years I was allowed to take care of a woman who, clinically speaking, was as ill as one could possibly be. She had undergone countless operations, suffered from metastatic sarcomas (a severe form of cancer), had dialysis-requiring kidney failure, had hepatitis C due to the many necessary blood washes, could hardly walk because of a chronic hip disorder, and was finally as good as blind. Medically she was a hopeless case – but as a human alive and hopeful. She always said – and I could believe her – that her illnesses were the greatest gift she had ever experienced. Otherwise, she would have continued to live the way she had done before without ever waking up. She had been professionally successful, had lived very independently, had had friends and partners, but lost herself completely. Now, with near death before her eyes, she enjoyed every minute and lived as intensely as never before. Was this woman sicker or healthier than before the onset of her symptoms? She herself had a completely different opinion from her doctors. She saw her 'diseases' as a successful attempt to heal her life – although she would die of them soon. In her suffering she had found a greater wholeness of self than before and a new attitude to life. Her relationships deepened and she was busy helping, counselling and comforting others. Her body was already damaged to such an extent that its integrity could not be restored, but Gisela lived with her newly won inner centre for five happy years despite a prognosis made out in a few weeks. – And I will always be grateful to her for the lesson she taught me about the values of life by being who she was.

This does not mean that obvious causes of disease should be denied. Conventional medicine is certainly right when it comes to naming the causes of diseases, viruses, bacteria, toxins, education, traumas, etc. But just as certainly this approach does not lead further when it comes to healing. Eliminating the cause of a disease is only useful in the long run if I consider disease (and therefore life itself) to be a meaningless event. Illness is then not the expression of something, but an unfortunate mishap that must be repaired. Dethlefsen and Dahlke go so far as to say: "Illness makes humans curable. Illness is the turning point at which disaster can be transformed into salvation. For this to happen, humans must stop fighting it and instead learn to hear and see what the disease has to say to them. The patient must listen within himself and communicate with his symptoms if he wants to experience their message. (...) So he must make the symptom superfluous by letting into consciousness what's wrong with him. Healing is always associated with an expansion of consciousness and maturation."[8]

When we seek such an approach to healing, there are three things to consider: First, consciousness has nothing to do with psychological interpretation. This is often confused. If I read somewhere or my therapist tells me what a certain symptom stands for, then I may have gained an interesting cognitive insight, but no greater consciousness and no more health. The interpretation of processes in life is often important in order to give them a place in our mental image of reality and thus also to calm the mind, but it does not change anything about reality itself. Awareness is something completely different. It arises when bright consciousness is brought into the symptom itself, which until then could only be experienced as pain or discomfort. Thus this symptom is reintegrated into the spiritual-mental-physical organism of the person and is usually brought back to the level from which it originated. Awareness means that we integrate 'what's wrong with us'. This process is conscious, but usually not verbal. Again and again I meet people who have been through long psychotherapies and can tell me precisely why they have their problems, what the causes are and why they have to express physically. But the problem, the cause of which you can now specify, still remains. An act of consciousness does not take place in the mind, but in the body. It is a typical confusion of our time to take the thinking and talking everyday consciousness for *the* consciousness. However, the parts of consciousness that are at stake in most diseases are not subject to mental access. Feeling is often one step closer to the level that matters, and sensation even more.

The second trap in this approach is the culturally deeply rooted guilt that starts immediately when it is determined that something has to do with me personally. Therefore, it seems to be an incredible relief for many people if an external diagnosis is found for their disease and if it

38

is not 'psychological'. Apart from the fact that the holistic view of homeopathy does not know this division into external and internal causes of illness, the whole approach has nothing to do with the attribution of guilt if one connects illness with one's own life and assumes responsibility for it.

Thirdly, the path of consciousness is one that many holistic therapists today favour, but which was initially not part of the homeopathic tradition. It is possible to heal people with no regard to their consciousness, i.e. to eliminate symptoms, without a connection to their life becoming clear to those concerned. In this respect, the disease with its symptoms is only an open offer to become conscious, not an obligation. However, being sick is one of the greatest learning opportunities that life offers us, precisely because personal suffering – unlike collective events – is very much tailored to us, the perfect mirror, so to speak, of 'what's wrong with us'. However, those people who have once embarked on the path of consciousness can no longer simply opt for 'unconscious' healing. Their symptoms inevitably urge for a conscious treatment.

When we think about illness having a point in human destiny and not preventing us, but rather contributing to our becoming 'whole' in a more comprehensive sense ("that our indwelling, rational mind can freely use this living, healthy tool for the higher purpose of our existence", as Hahnemann puts it[9]), then these thoughts only apply to those circumstances of life under which individual destiny can be realised at all. Where people live in total misery, as we unfortunately allow a large part of humanity to do, tormented by plagues and famines, it is pointless to speak of illness as a way or a task of destiny for the individual. Individual meaning can only be made accessible where the individual is sufficiently free from the collective forces to be able to deal with one's own experience of fate at all. In such circumstances, humanity as a whole is the diseased organism that has to learn and find a new balance. The special thing about human life is that we are always carrying and enduring meaning on several levels at once: as individuals, as part of families and ancestral lines, as part of larger social movements, as part of peoples and nations, as part of religious movements and finally as part of humanity.

For a deeper understanding of our lives it is crucial to ask the question of meaning on the proper level. The experiences with family constellations and systemic therapy in recent years have made it clear to what extent a family destiny can have impact on an individual person 'without regard for the personality', so to speak. Certain experiences of fate in an individual can almost be predicted solely from the position in the line of ancestors and in the family system, independent of the personal characteristics and inclinations of the individual concerned. For us as individualists this notion can be very disturbing.

Homeopathic theory has anticipated these findings with the idea of miasms, which cross generations and determine the disposition to certain types of disease. Without a healing of these 'miasms' – according to Hahnemann – lasting health is not possible, not even with good individual treatment according to the law of similarity. The miasm theory has remained controversial among homeopaths, because in it Hahnemann subordinated pure observation to a theory and, on top of that, did not elaborate it in a particularly plausible way. In any case, every homeopath seems to understand it differently.

When it comes to questions about the meaningfulness of illness, the understanding of health, the relationship between collective and individual processes, we move beyond empiricism in the field of speculation and world view. When I ask about the meaning of illness and health, I also have to ask what meaning I want to give to life at all. Every healing method that takes itself seriously demands this discussion. The questions are answered again and again, by every therapist, every sufferer, every generation, every culture. It is important to keep in mind that every attempted answer to the question of meaning always precedes the decision for a healing method and can never be empirically justified.

The individual answers are never detached from the ideological, philosophical or religious framework from which their language, imagery and structure originate. In the following chapters we will look at the mental concepts of homeopathy. And this will also show the significance that the underlying philosophy has regarding the use of homeopathy as a healing method for our lives, because this is the true fascination of homeopathy for all those who have come closer to it.

40

Dynamis – the Life Force

All homeopathic students first learn that this healing method works by influencing the life force according to the law of similarity. They then spend some years learning more about the law of similarity and its application, but with regard to the life force there just remains the vague notion that it is 'out of tune' during illness and must be brought back into balance correctly for recovery.

But what exactly the life force is, what qualities it has and what laws it is subject to, remains open, the question is not even posed.

At least I want to try the latter here: to ask the question as to what we can imagine about the 'life force' and to suggest a few approaches to an understanding. To put it bluntly: in this chapter there are no answers, only questions, approaches, reflections. If, however, the vital force as the central idea of homeopathy comes into view in a new way, then the chapter has reached its goal.

First of all, it is noticeable that the views on what is meant by the term already diverge as widely as possible.

Hahnemann helped to create this problem in so far as he expects us to accept a complex theoretical construction ("illness is based solely on a derangement of the spiritual life force"), about which he simultaneously imposes a prohibition of thought ("no speculations and brooding") and which he himself uses contradictorily in the *Organon* (cf. §§9 and 288-89).

If the question of life force is not only considered as a matter of homeopathic history but also as a question of what constitutes life as life, the question leads us into the midst of today's most sensitive topics of philosophy – and into the midst of the basic philosophical question about the origin and constitution of humanity itself. The questions about the origin and the basic conditions of our being and existence belong to the field of metaphysics, ontology – a part of philosophy that has become increasingly taboo in the course of modern times, since all questions about what goes beyond the empirical, sensual experience of everyday, 'normal' human beings and does not directly serve the practical problems of action, is often considered inadmissible.

Nevertheless, for many of us a concept of what constitutes the life force can be experienced in real life and can be felt and sensed as vitality, as an energy flow. Generally 'life' is in a way similar to the concept of time of which Augustine says: "So what is time? If no one asks me about it, I know it, but if I should explain it to someone who asks me, I don't know it;"[10]

The question of 'life force' uses the terms 'life' and 'force'.

Last but not least, this holistic approach of 'life force – animated organism – wholeness' touches the ancient body and soul problem, i.e. the interaction of body and mind, matter and spirit. Also the definition of health and illness (see *Organon* §9; illness as a derangement of the life force; health as being whole, healing as 'whole being') is connected with the topic.

As a first approximation, three different positions can be distinguished:

a)   Vitality is an abstract, holistic concept. Historically and philosophically this approach is called 'vitalism'.
b)   Life force is a concrete agent that is subject to certain laws and can also be quantified.
c)   Life force is a superfluous concept; the term does not denote reality and should be abandoned. A systems-theoretical concept helps us more in understanding homeopathic effects.

Susanne Diez has dealt extensively with point a) in an article in *Documenta Homeopathica*.[11]

Point c), which is not discussed in this chapter, is represented with excellent reasoning by Georg Ivanovas[12]. Even if this point of view will be rejected by some classical homeopaths, (and I don't share it either) the positions are well worth considering and point to some weak points of the life force concept. In dialogue with a positivistic approach to science of the conventional paradigm, we will not be able to avoid dealing in detail and constructively with this point of view and appreciating its strengths.

42

Point b) is less a philosophical question than a pragmatic one. This approach will be the subject of this chapter.[13]

If we want to deal with the life force, then it makes sense to extend our view to other fields of knowledge, in which a lot of knowledge has already collected. What can we learn from the concept of the flow of *chi* in the meridians of the body used by Chinese medicine for millennia? Is this *chi* our *dynamis*, or something like that, or not comparable? If we take our own concepts seriously, we cannot avoid such questions. And what about the orgone of Reichian Psychodynamics?

And above all: What are our own experiences in healing with the life force?

Surprisingly, this is hardly thought of at all. I know significantly more texts on antidotes or other side issues than considerations of what it means exactly to influence life force. Hahnemann has already shown us a way in this direction: In his §§288-89 on Mesmerism, he deals with the question of how this power can be transferred directly from person to person. So he is obviously not interested in an abstract concept, as if the 'dynamic derangement' could also be replaced by another theorem. Rather, he regards the life force as a fact which is not physical but 'spiritual', yet very real, to which the physical processes are subordinated and which can be influenced in different ways.

When Hahnemann writes in the first fundamental sections of his *Organon* (§§9-11) about the life force, he seems to point to a general principle to be understood philosophically: "The material organism, thought without life force, is not capable of any sensation, any activity, any self-preservation; only the immaterial being invigorating the material organism in the healthy and sick state (the life principle, the life force) gives it all sensation and effects its life directions."(§10) However, if we look at the §§ in which he writes concretely and practically, for example about Mesmerism (§§288-89), it becomes clear that he rather imagines a non-material, but quite concrete and transferable fluidum. Otherwise it cannot be understood that he talks about the inflow and outflow of the life force, about its lack or surplus and about the transfer from one human being to another. In his "Versuch über ein neues Prinzip zur Auffindung der Heilkräfte der Arzneisubstanzen [Search for a new principle of the healing properties of drug substances]" (p.137) he even speaks of "the area of the stomach (the area of the presumed main organ of the life force)", thus sees the life force as localised in the body and provided with a recognisable structure. Reading of the 'main organ' of the life force we are tempted to think of the chakras of the Hindu and Buddhist image of the human energetic body[14].

In general, it could be a worthwhile project to consider the organisation of the life force in the human organism in the form of chakras or meridians for homeopathic theory as well. On the one hand, this would make it easier to differentiate the understanding of life force from a homeopathic point of view. On the other hand, this understanding could serve as a bridge to other holistic methods such as TCM or Ayurveda, to bioenergetic therapies and spiritual healing methods, the findings and diagnoses of which can hardly be translated into homeopathic terms hitherto.

How can we form an idea or model of how the patterns we try to describe with homeopathic remedies and the amount of this life force itself interact to health? And what is the relationship between Hahnemann's concept of the *dynamis* and the other medical systems mentioned?

I would like to propose here a model that combines two different therapeutic approaches to the life force and points to some interesting practical consequences. As with everything that comes into existence, we can distinguish two aspects of the life force: the content and the form, here called more precisely the pure energy and the structure or the pattern. Although the formation of the term 'vital force' suggests that it is only about the pure force aspect, its use shows that this is not the case. If different homeopathic remedies have different effects, then we are dealing with a differentiation that lies in the structure, unless we want to accept an infinite number of completely different 'life forces'. But since 'life force' is only used in the singular, we can assume a distinction into the mere force and its structure: just as a sound has an aspect of pure energy that lies in the mere intensity of air movement and an aspect of structure that lies in the frequency and distribution of overtones. A sound is on the one hand a physical force (air movement) that can also be transformed into heat or electricity, and on the other

44

hand information that can be written down as a note or burned onto a CD as a digital pattern. If I look only at the physical energy component, there is no difference between music and noise, which lacks information. If I look only at the written notes, I have only the information without physical expression. I can only hear a song if both are present.

The Western forms of therapy based on life force have so far addressed both aspects separately – in contrast to Chinese and Indian medicine, which consider both at the same time.[15] Mesmerism, spiritual healers, and Reich therapists[16] are predominantly concerned with the purely quantitative aspect of life force, while homeopathy focuses entirely on the aspect of information by trying to influence the pattern in which energy is processed. Hahnemann himself, as already mentioned, had in mind to increase the amount of vital energy, or to release it and to influence it favourably by extensive dietary measures. However, these approaches have hardly been taken up by his successors and no longer play a real role today.

The forms of therapy of Wilhelm Reich's followers and the resulting body therapies approach the problem more from the energy side and rely on the fact that a sufficient amount of free-flowing life energy is bound to restore health on its own.[17]

Another word about the term 'energy': It is common in modern homeopathy to speak of the homeopathic remedies as transmitting 'energy' or 'vibrations'. This word use does not make sense, because what we detach from the initial material substance of our remedy and imprint on the carrier medium (alcohol, sugar, water) by potentisation is information. If we imagine globules as carriers of energy, they would be a kind of small battery, and the thicker the globule, the greater their energy would have to be, because energy can be multiplied. And they would lose energy to the environment over time and have a fixed expiry date. We know that none of this is the case. The homeopathic medicine therefore does not transfer 'energy', but information, a pattern. So it doesn't matter whether the globules are big or small, whether I take one or three and whether I take sugar pellets or alcohol drops, just as it doesn't matter whether I print a poem on a big or small sheet or write it on the table or copy it five times. The information remains the same; at most its accessibility is influenced.

If we look at this splitting of the life force into the aspects of force (energy, content) and structure (pattern, form), as it is typical for homeopathy in Hahnemann's sense, it is easy to understand why Hahnemann in all his writings describes the life force as 'instinctive, mindless and unconscious' and does not believe that the body controlled by it has the power to heal itself. As long as the life force is imagined as separated from its information, then it is 'mindless' and we have to imprint the information, the pattern, on it with the help of remedies. Self-healing only works if both are true: If there is sufficient basic strength available and if the effective pattern fits the problem. To make a technical comparison: the best computer programme does not work if there is no electricity, but a lot of electricity does not do the job by itself either if the wrong programme is switched on.

However, this division is an artificial, purely conceptual one. In reality, both aspects usually occur together. As little as I can split a song into the 'mindless' air pressure and the notes, as little is there a mere instinctive life force in the body that can only receive its information through globules.

But it can well happen that I play a song too quietly or too loudly and therefore it cannot be perceived properly. And it can also be that I play it wrong, and then it doesn't sound better if I turn the volume way up. According to this model I would try to understand the influence of different therapeutic measures on the life force.

With our different potencies we already have a certain mechanism to put the information given into the organism 'loudly' or 'quietly' – even if there are as many theories as homeopaths about the respective use of the potencies. And we also hear that in very weakened patients we should be 'careful' with the administration of remedies, because the vital force is so low that a reaction to the remedy is difficult to cope with. But how do I give a remedy 'carefully'? When are remedies 'loud' or 'quiet'? There are no clear ideas about that. Hahnemann would have said: 'quiet' or 'careful' are potencies as high as possible, because they reduce the toxicity and the remedy affects the body in a more subtle way. Today, many homeopaths would say that low potencies are 'cautious' because they are less intensive. So what? – We notice that there is no theory on the subject on the basis of which we can order the observations meaningfully and draw conclusions from them.

If we knew more about the laws of the life force, we would be able to recognise states of its quantitative deficiency (in distinction to mere misdirection of its pattern) and – in addition to the application of remedies – accelerate a healing process through targeted supply or stimulation (as apparently Hahnemann did). In general, we have an idea of what is beneficial to the amount of vitality: a healthy diet, exercise in the fresh air, a good rhythm of work and relaxation, emotional security, etc. But what exactly is it? Is it true, for example, that modern denatured food contains sufficient chemical substances, but too little vital energy? Or that the life force is more present in fresh raw food than in cooked food? Are there really places with concentrated life force ('power places') where the organism can 'charge' itself? Or 'overload'? About all this there is a lot of knowledge that we homeopaths don't have and might well need. But there are also a lot of superstitions and ideologies that we don't need. It will take great effort to separate the wheat from the chaff and to separate real knowledge from wishes and fantasies. Yet it is necessary.

An essential aspect of this understanding of the life force is that in principle it should be perceptible and there are a number of people who claim to be able to perceive it directly and that such perceptions are learnable. For we homeopaths it would of course be an immeasurable advantage to be able to 'see' or 'sense' the vital force directly and thus also to be able to judge our interventions with homeopathic remedies not only indirectly and interpretively on the basis of the changes in the symptoms, but directly. It is therefore astonishing that there are no more efforts to explore this area in an unbiased way. Apparently, the smell of the 'esoteric' that emanates from these issues is so repulsive that it is best to avoid such ideas, no matter how obviously important they are when considered soberly.

What practical consequences could these considerations have in therapeutic work? Let's take a patient with minor constitutional weaknesses, but without serious illnesses. In damp and cold weather he notices his knee joints under strain and in emotional tension and pressure at work his stomach hurts and he gets heartburn. After the holidays and after long weekends, this person is symptom-free and feels healthy. A longer fasting cure and the change to a less stressful job had the same effect. However, any prolonged exposure would cause the symptoms to return. – This is a typical picture, often seen in practice, which means that as the overall level of vital energy increases, existing structural weaknesses do not appear, are not perceived. The patient feels 'healthy.' If the level of the life force decreases, the same problems occur again and again, like undersea mountains, which become visible each time the water level sinks.

Now there are two different approaches to healing. As a homeopath I would try to influence the structure by recognising its pattern and neutralising it. If I succeed in this completely, the symptom should no longer occur, regardless of the level of my life force or perception. This means that even when the level drops, no peaks become visible, and I remain symptom-free. As an energetic healer, however, I would try to raise the level of the life force so that existing weaknesses no longer appear.

Within the framework of this model, the strengths and weaknesses of both approaches are obvious. If the level of power falls far enough, new disturbance patterns will appear again and again even after the elimination of the main problems, because even with the best homeopathic remedies no perfect human beings can be created. If I only raise the vital level again and again and leave the problematic patterns in the processing of the life force untouched, it will quickly sink again and the energetic healing will become a Sisyphean task. In fact, it would be optimal to consider both aspects (as Hahnemann did). If we were to acquire as much exact knowledge about the energy aspect of the life force as we have about its patterns, we would have an even safer healing method at our disposal.

Another Reality

The founder of homeopathy gave much importance to the approach of homeopathy not being a world view, but a healing method or art of healing. And this is how most homeopaths see it up until the present day. Something is right about that, because a medical system alone cannot represent a world view. On the other hand, however, *every* way of healing – like every other method or knowledge – stands within the framework of a certain world view, a paradigm, thus a comprehensive interpretation of reality, which gives meaning and context to its theses and its actions.

One of the main problems persons and therapists interested in homeopathy meet is that the mode of action of homeopathic remedies is not explained and that their therapeutic action is not embedded in any comprehensive theory of the world. Even practising homeopaths often cannot give a good theory for their actions, at least not one that would stand up to some scrutiny. The experiences made with homeopathy as well as its rules seem to stand in an ideological void and have no recognisable connection to our current view of the world.

A principle such as the law of similarity is hardly more than a mere assertion if it has its place within the framework of an order that promises to explain a larger section of the world than the process of healing. Without such a background – conscious or unconscious – we can neither understand nor meaningfully apply the guidelines of a healing method. **An holistic medicine must be part of an holistic science within the framework of a corresponding world view**, just as conventional medicine is part of the mechanistic sciences and the positivistic-materialistic world view.

With regard to homeopathic healing there is often talk of 'energies' and 'vibrations', but these terms only sound as if they could explain something, since they do not refer to physically defined vibrations or forces. These terms do not point to known things, but introduce mysterious new qualities for explanation, which are meant to remind us of physical terms. It is also difficult to refer to scientific studies on homeopathy, of which there are many, since these studies can scientifically prove the existence of homeopathic effects in principle[18]. However, with their help nothing can be said about the complex homeopathic laws.[19]

Many patients who are otherwise critical and well-informed about treatments and practitioners accept that homeopathy is not transparent for them in terms of both the way it works and the strategy of treatment. On the one hand, this shows that confidence in alternative methods is not as drastically lost as in conventional medicine. On the other hand, the holistic approach and the search for similarity seem to meet with an intuitive resonance even without a valid theory. Homeopathy is obviously linked to an intuitive basic understanding of humans and the world. But a conscious and responsible decision for a form of therapy is only possible if the philosophical or scientific backgrounds can be reflected and processed.

Homeopathy can reasonably be explained and brought into a clear theoretical context, but not within the framework of mechanistic, materialistic or physicalistic science.

In the historical development of homeopathy it was fatal that at Hahnemann's time there was no suitable explanatory framework available for homeopathy. For the world view into which homeopathy fits seamlessly is the so-called *hermetic*, or as we would say today, the *esoteric*[20]. This had lost its formative power in the West in the century before Hahnemann and was considered unworthy of discussion in Hahnemann's medical and social circles. He would therefore not have been able to fall back on it even if he had been aware of the connection. For him it was self-evident to lean on the explanatory structures of rational Enlightenment and to build up his system in the sense of the sciences that were currently developing then. His idea of developing a medicine that could achieve the precision of mathematics is naive, measured by our contemporary knowledge of humans, but understandable from the pathos of Enlightenment of his time. At his time, Hahnemann could not yet know that the mechanistic sciences would not be able to provide a useful theoretical model for homeopathy even in their heyday. Just before the time when homeopathy came into being the world view to which it belongs had just gone out of fashion, yet Hahnemann was able to fall back on a kind of intuitive a priori understanding on the part of his contemporaries. Otherwise, his therapeutic approach would not have found acceptance anywhere.

In order to understand the juxtaposition of world views that has been made here, one must realise that our habitual idea, that the mechanistic sciences provide an 'objective' or true view of the world, is wrong. Every view and interpretation of our perceptions of the world can only be one of several possible ones. Any interpretation of the world, or as modern theory of science puts it: any *paradigm*, proceeds from certain unprovable presuppositions – the axioms – which distinguish it from other world views and lead to a specific view of things. The mechanistic sciences describe in their own way a certain view of the world, just as other philosophies describe equally valuable yet different views of the world. Each of them sets the limits of the world and of what is possible in a different place; for each world view different processes are understandable or impossible. Each has different ideas of time and space, subjective and objective, spirit and matter, as well as other values following from these basic assumptions.[21] These reasons are in principle not provable and cannot be wrong or right, because they form the logical basis to which everything else is traced back, but which itself can no longer be traced back to anything. This applies equally to all paradigms.

It is customary for every cultural epoch to have a particular world view, dominant in its time, which is regarded as 'the truth' – one also speaks of the prevailing paradigm. This dominant world view changes with time. In recent decades, for example, it has been observed within the Euro-American cultural sphere that the consensus on the 'objectivity' of the scientific world view that had been valid for two hundred years has been shaken. (See the final chapter for details.) We are in a period of cultural transition in which it becomes clear that there can be several valid systems and traditions of thinking about the world, under which the materialistic sciences of western complexion represent one possibility only. The fact that the mechanistic concept of faith is developing distinctly fundamentalist forms in 2019, which will be discussed in detail in a later chapter, and on the basis of which an ideological roll-back into the 19th century is attempted, cannot hide the fact that the idea of being able to comprehend the world and its living beings as machines is finally outdated and will not come again.

What is that world view, from which homeopathy can be derived and explained well? What does homeopathy have in common with alchemy and shamanism that I can name it in one breath? We refer to a world view with which humanity has lived, and still lives, for hundreds of thousands of years all over the world. For those of us who have grown up in the mental habits of rationalism and scientism, it is usually difficult to imagine that the world view that seems natural and 'objective' to us is only a fleeting fad in world history. Since the modern world view does not aim to *understand* the world, but to measure, calculate and manipulate it, it has created incredible instruments of power (technical as well as social) in the shortest possible time to bring nature and people under its control worldwide. Although it is barely two hundred years old and understood by most people in fragments only, it has been predominant on this planet for a many decades. It is a very one-sided and therefore probably temporary phenomenon, which will gradually (and hopefully without major catastrophes) give way to a more comprehensive image of the world and of man, and integrate itself into an holistic world view. The peak of the rationalist-scientist phase has already passed, and we are experiencing the downside everywhere. It is no coincidence that medicine is the source of impulses to question the superficial view of mechanistic science. In the middle of the last century, when scientism seemed to have gained autocracy, when all hopes were directed towards ever better technology and ever more chemistry, and when even the theologians said goodbye to God and the soul, it was only occultism and alternative medicine that preserved the remains of a holistic view of the world. Since the eighties the sheet has gradually changed so that today it is possible to openly present the ideological foundations of a medical direction such as homeopathy without publicly disqualifying oneself. The time of improper and also ineffective ingratiation with the mechanistic way of thinking is over.

Today we are confronted with the task to get to know the old (and new) world view again and to open ourselves to its perspective and approach. What are the characteristic features and what are the spiritual pillars on which it is based? And how does homeopathy fit into this *philosophia perennis*, into eternal wisdom? – That is the subject of this chapter.

The World View of the Ancient World

All peoples have always lived in a world which the Greeks called '*Cosmos*': a meaningfully ordered world in contrast to *Chaos* (the world of randomness and arbitrariness into which we are thrown in modernity). In a *Cosmos* all beings and things have their place and their meaning. Everything is connected with everything else; interrelated and referring to everything. Everything is alive and animate, from stones to the gods. And the different layers of existence are experienced as permeable; the spiritual is not strictly separated from the physical: the world a great and complex unity.

Over endless periods of human history this world view found its expression in myth, the last traces of which have come to us in fairy tales. The mythical world shows itself in the most different of pictures, but its depth is the same everywhere in the world. In mythology, the knowledge of the world is combined with the knowledge of the soul – psychology and cosmology are identical.

Only two and a half thousand years ago, with the ancient Greeks, did the European people begin a special path. The consciousness of the individual human being began to face the world in a new way, to ask new questions and to feel estranged. The unified culture disintegrated into different aspects: politics, religion, philosophy, magic, science, medicine, art – a movement that consistently led to our specialisation. Until then, healing and spirituality, the knowledge of fate and the body, herbalism and rituals were inseparable units of one life.

Of the various emerging traditions, some carried with them for longer than others the old knowledge and remnants of the old way of life. These traditions – among them magic, astrology, alchemy and medicine – migrated over the centuries into the cultural underground and preserved the old, holistic view of reality, often though in a diffuse or even distorted way. After the legendary sage Hermes Trismegistos, the thrice largest Hermes, who bears the name of the Greek messenger of the gods and guide of the dead, it was long referred to as *hermeticism*. In the European Middle Ages it was long regarded as *scientia*, as science as such, then carried the names of Hermetism or occultism in the high time of materialism, and today it is mostly called esotericism.

In some respects alchemy is most similar to homeopathy and unites essential features of the old world view up to practical application. Alchemy gathered all the ancient knowledge about nature, minerals and plants, and had a direct relation to medicine and produced its own remedies.

Alchemy

Among the great ancient traditions, alchemy can probably claim the highest age. It reaches far into mythical times and can be traced back to the oldest human efforts to influence matter.[22] When humans learned to work the metals, they saw this as an intervention in the course of nature, as the touching of a mystery. From the beginning, blacksmiths were considered magicians whose work was surrounded by taboos and often twilight[23] because it was connected with the interior of matter and the mysteriously transforming fire. Prometheus, who brought fire to men, was cruelly punished by the gods for it. Among the Teutons, certain dwarves, the black elves, were in possession of the art of blacksmithing. They were rich and clever, but unpredictable and insidious. Even today, we associate the devil with fire and the smell of sulphur. Sulphur, however, was one of the three alchemical basic elements (Mercury, Sulphur and Salt).

The archaic conception of the world, which survived in alchemy, was based on living matter that matured and grew in the womb of the earth mother. This maturation of matter could be accelerated by suitable actions accompanied by rituals. Metals could be transformed and coloured. The alchemist wanted to lift matter to the highest level of being, which was symbolised by the metal 'gold'. This process went hand in hand with the spiritual maturation of the alchemist, who there-

54

Already in ancient times alchemy was closely related to the neoplatonic-gnostic thoughts about the ascent and descent of the soul and together with these formed the basis of so-called hermeticism. The hermetic-alchemistic writings that gave this tradition its name were written in the first centuries by neo-platonic Gnostics. The Corpus Hermeticum bears the name of the god Hermes, the Greek messenger of the gods and master of science and magic. Very clearly these representations are marked as contents of mental experiences and thus are distinguished from merely theoretical speculations. For centuries esoterics and alchemists referred to this literature. Until modern times, science and magic were regarded as one. '*Scientia*", as science was also called at the later universities, was either astrology or *magia naturalis,* the natural magic.

After antiquity followed the dark centuries of the early Middle Ages, in which the Roman Empire disintegrated, Christianity spread in Europe and various Germanic princely houses fought for supremacy; the 'Dark Ages' as the English say, in which culturally almost nothing moved. European culture only flourished again in the 11th and 12th centuries in scholasticism and mysticism. Through Arab mediation, Aristotle returned to the Western European world. But not only classical scholarship, but also the occult arts were revived by the Arab influence. The names *alchemy, alcohol, alkahest* and others already show the Arabic influence on alchemy. It was not until the Renaissance that the European horizon really opened up again to the Greek heritage in its many mythological and esoteric aspects. What stood in contrast to the established view of the world at that time, however, are not those aspects that seem esoteric, occult or strange to us today. Today we would call the entire world view of European Christianity at that time magical or esoteric. On the contrary, modernity was a thorn in the side of the church's renaissance, the spiritual power that dominated everything at that time. Many great spirits began to search for truth independently and free from ecclesiastical authority, not confining themselves to the Bible. This spiritual wrestling has been investigated and described many times. Little known — but essential for understanding modern times — is the fact that many of the philosophers, artists and scientists of the Renaissance and subsequent periods were hermetics and alchemists: Pico de la Mirandola, Paracelsus, Giordano Bruno, John Dee, Isaac Newton, Francis Bacon, to name but a few. The focus of intellectual interests shifted more and more from speculation and interpretation of the classics to self-gained experience. This can already be measured by the high number of printed alchemy books, which was around 1600 at 150 editions per year with about 75000 to 120000 copies, which is a surprisingly high number for the time of the invention of the printing machine.[24]

Of course, the many recipes for making gold and preparing the elixir of life led countless adventurers to try and make a profit out of it. It is clear that their chemical success was low. Often, however, they had considerable success with princes who allowed themselves to be talked into miracles for a lot of money.

Alchemy was, and is often, regarded as fraudulent 'gold making'. But already since the 14th century B.C. the chemical gold test was known, which made falsifications and fraud at the very least, risky. A transformation of the metals into one another was considered possible, since matter was regarded as a unit, as alive, and in constant slow transformation. But already from ancient texts it is clear that the alchemists had another, religious goal in mind. This applies to Indian and Chinese alchemy as[25] well as to Western alchemy. In general, the alchemists' interest in chemistry in our sense was rather low. From an alchemical point of view, modern chemistry cannot be regarded as a successor, but only as a sad product of decay. The alchemists were as little interested in chemistry as the Freemasons were in building houses. C.G. Jung points out that instead alchemical work was often accompanied by visions and dreams that were given great value.

by attained immortality. The alchemical laboratory work was prayer, meditation and experiment in one.

With the deconsecration of the material world, which was prepared by Christianity and carried out by scientific ideology to the last possible consequence, alchemy lost its effectiveness as a path of spiritual realisation. Chemistry adopted some of its methods and used them for completely different purposes. Its symbols were partly spiritualised and partly lost.

56

It was C.G. Jung who, in this century, once again drew attention to the fact that alchemy was more than just primitive chemistry under erroneous conditions.[26] In detailed studies he proved the initiation path (Jung calls it individuation) of the alchemist in contact with his 'matter'. This alchemical view of matter is hardly comprehensible for modern man. After all, most people find it difficult enough to visualise the divine in the execution of communion. "One need only imagine a communion that would no longer be confined to the figures of bread and wine, but would be extended to the contact with each 'substance' in order to measure the distance that exists between such an archaic religious experience and the modern experience of the 'natural phenomena'".[27]

But since we cannot simply step out of our way of experiencing nature today, and since alchemy is a path of inner and outer experience intimately connected, it can hardly be revived today. Apart from a few exceptions,[28] this term today refers either to a kind of para-chemistry or to imaginative methods based on Jung.[29]

Yet in homeopathy we find, throughout the entire development of modernity, a well functioning and practically applied reminder of this view of the world as living, coherent and meaningful. Homeopathy still practises in its own way the dissolution of matter through a sophisticated ritual, into a spiritual essence that is symbolically bound to an agent (water, sugar, alcohol) but does not therein exhaust its existence.

In ancient times, in Alexandria from the second century B.C. to the second century A.D. western alchemy took on the forms that remained until modern times. In the sacred mysteries of that epoch, the initiates experienced the death and resurrection of the God (Dionysus, Iakchos, Mithras, Jesus) in the form of a mythical drama. The alchemist, on the other hand, experienced the descent and ascent of his or her soul in the image of changing matter, which underwent the phases of dissolution, purification, maturation and perfection in the laboratory – a tremendous material-psychical-spiritual process, which the alchemists called 'the Great Work'. The associated images[30] strongly recall shamanic initiation rites and visions in which the initiates experienced their dismemberment, death and resurrection in the flesh.

It is important to realise that the alchemists did not experience these processes as a symbolic 'as-if'. For them, the material process was really[31] connected to their spiritual life in a way that we can hardly imagine today. They were aware of the paradox of this relationship when, for example, about the philosopher's stone, the elixir or the philosophical gold it was written that it was not ordinary gold and could be found everywhere on the street, but nobody recognised it. On the other hand, considerable precautions were taken to ensure that no one learned the 'secret' of how to make gold or stone. This led to the fact that alchemical texts in their encoding are hardly understandable for later and uninitiated readers. Autodidacts were denied access via reading. Only the initiation by a master of alchemy granted access to the art of the arts. For not only spiritual contents were described chemically, but also chemical substances and processes in reverse with mythical images, which made the confusion complete.

In practice, the alchemists proceeded in such a way that they first returned matter to its original state and thus won the *materia prima,* from which all other states could be obtained by maturing processes. The highest attainable state of matter was considered the philosopher's stone or *lapis philosophorum.* With the preparation of the Philosopher's Stone, the alchemists reached a mystical goal with which they approached cosmic unity again. Even if the procedure, the goal and the imagery of alchemy may seem irrational to us, they are based on an understandable, rational and coherent structure. It shares this structure with homeopathy, as we will explain later.

Since salvation and healing are close to each other (in German: *Heil* and *Heilung*), the alchemists have also dealt with the healing and alleviation of physical ailments and illnesses, and in some cases even placed this at the centre of their work. "Indian and Chinese alchemy focused on the production of life-prolonging preparations, while Western alchemy was more interested in the transmutation of metals.[32] But also in Europe a tradition of the alchemical preparation of medicines developed, which are known as 'spagyric' and still exist today. Such medicines, also known as 'Arcana', can be obtained from a number of specialised laboratories.

Apart from the individual remedies for certain ailments, in the Arcana, there was also the idea of a panacea, the 'Panacée', or the elixir, a substance that would be able to heal any ailment on the spot and give physical immortality to those who possessed it. Numerous are the stories about adepts who survived centuries and appeared under different names. There is a number of well-documented healing accounts (including one by Goethe about a mysterious alchemical healing in himself, which justified his lifelong interest in this discipline) which suggest that the stories handed down had a true core beyond their legendary form, and told of healing arts based on a targeted transformation of matter and seemed like miracles to contemporaries.

The individual spagyric remedies are in the same relationship to the elixir as the individual metal transformations are to the Great Work. Thus one can perhaps distinguish between alchemical works of lower and higher order. The production of the Philosopher's Stone, the Great Work and the production of the Elixir are therefore often regarded as a single process. Only the entirely mature adept can obtain the elixir. Only he (or she) has mastered the microcosm, purified their own soul and allowed it to mature, and can thus also exert a comprehensive influence on the macrocosm. Thus it corresponds to the laws of the analogy of microcosm and macrocosm, of above and below, of inside and outside.

The Tabula Smaragdina (the *Emerald Tablet*).

It is true without lying, certain and most true.
That which is below is like that which is above
and that which is above is like that which is below
to do the miracles of one only thing.
And as all things have been and arose from one by the meditation
of the one: so all things have their birth from this one thing by
analogy.
The Sun is its father, the Moon its mother, the wind has carried it
in its belly, the earth is its nurse.
This is the father of all the perfection of the world.
Its power is entire if it be converted into earth.
Separate thou the earth from the fire, the subtle from the gross
sweetly with great industry.
It ascends from the earth to the heaven and again it descends to
the earth and receives the force of things superior and inferior.
By this means you shall have the glory of the whole world
and thereby all obscurity shall fly from you.
Its force is above all force, for it vanquishes every subtle thing
and penetrates every solid thing.
So was the world created.
From this are and do come admirable adaptations,
whereof the means is here in this.
Hence I am called Hermes Trismegistos,
holding the three parts of the philosophy of the whole world.
That which I have said of the operation of the Sun is
accomplished and ended. [33]

Micro- and Macrocosmos

The world of the ancient peoples has always been an orderly one, a great whole in which everything is animated and ensouled and connected in depth. Everything follows eternal laws that order our cosmos and make it a meaningful world in which every being has its place. However, the laws of this cosmos are different from what we now call the laws of nature, which are able to explain to us in detail the functioning of different material entities. To some extent, these cosmic laws found their expression in myths and fairy tales, in images whose meaning our modern thinking has yet to grasp, but which are still directly comprehensible to intuitive people, children and artists. Some of the laws were also explicitly formulated. However, the classical formulations of these laws, such as the famous emerald tablet (see box), are difficult for us to understand. Therefore, I will explain the Basic Laws in our terms.[34]

The basic laws of hermeticism, of the *Philosophia perennis,* the 'eternal philosophy', alchemy, magic or esotericism can be summarised as the *law of analogy,* the *law of polarity,* the *law of the levels of existence,* the *law of the mandala* and the *law of unity.* First the basics are explained and later the connection to homeopathy.

A pivotal role in this other reality is taken by *the law of analogy,* the correspondence of microcosm and macrocosm. The 'microcosm' here refers to the individual and the 'macrocosm' to the entire world. And the basic idea is that the macrocosm ("above") and the microcosm ("below") correspond to each other, which means that they refer to each other in a meaningful way – in modern terms, as in a holography, for example, where each fragment is a complete picture of the whole. This order is often summarised in the ancient sentence "As above, so below" and brings the universal connectedness of all things to one point.

"But also in what is generally called 'a coincidence' or in situations that repeat themselves in life, we encounter the law of similarity. Here we can follow what C.G. Jung says when he says that we encounter on the outside what we do not want to accept on the inside. (...) At this point it is important to realise that this law of similarity is not a random product of a healing art, but a universal law of relationship."[35]

For scientific thinkers of the materialistic habit it may seem unfamiliar that connectedness follows the rules of images and not those of material contact. An example: We can all probably follow the notion that the feeling of rage matches the colour red, perhaps even that the planet Mars has something to do with rage, since it is named after the god of war and is also called the red planet. All this seems spontaneously 'appropriate' to us. But that the planet Jupiter, the colour blue and the number 4 have the same connection with each other is not familiar to us. Just as we must learn to calculate and read so that series of numbers and letters make sense to us, we must also learn the laws of analogies before they make sense to us and before we can deal with them and apply them. This learning process takes place in most cultures through narratives and rituals; it permeates the whole world view, from religion to medicine to superstition.

For our contemporary, rather psychologically oriented understanding it is decisive that such an analogy relationship also exists from the inside of the human being to the outer world. Indeed, this modern distinction between 'inside' and 'outside' basically does not exist. There is only one world in which everything is connected, even through the different layers or levels of being. 'Above' and 'below' originally denoted the plane of the stars and the earthly world of the people who are in such an analogy relationship. In many contemporary discussions about astrology it is noticeable how little these principles are still understood today. There is always an argument about the possible effects of planets and stars on humans in order to prove or refute the astrological claims. But it is not at all about effects; these have – if they exist (like for example the causation of ebb and flow by the moon) – in any case nothing to do with astrology.[36] Analogy implies that all things in the cosmos (and exactly that makes up a *cosmos*) behave in meaningful correspondence to each other. That I am a choleric person, spontaneous and prone to outbursts of rage, and that the planet Mars is on my ascendant, have no causal connection to each other. Mars doesn't affect me in any way, but the position of this planet *matches* my character, Mars *matches* me. You could say that the planets demark certain qualities of time, like the arms of a clock demark the hours of a day, but they don't influence time in any way.

An important aspect of the old hermetic (and thus also homeopathic) way of thinking, which is important for medical thinking and procedure, is that there is no separation of body and soul. Everything is contained in everything and affects everything, microcosm and macrocosm correspond, all being has aspects or layers which we describe as physical, mental and spiritual, but there is no separation between a purely material body and a non-material soul, whose effects on each other would need explanation and strictly speaking cannot be explained.[37] The necessary division of healing into a mechanistic body medicine, a bodiless psychology and its patching together in 'psychosomatics' is not necessary and not meaningful from the holistic point of view described here, because in real life the physical, the mental and the spiritual occur as a unity. The body-soul problem will not be solved by finding out how the soul can affect the body. By definition, it could do this only by overriding the laws of nature, which are formulated without a mental component. The solution can only lie in starting from a view of the world that does not make such a division, but orients itself on the experienced reality in which the world forms a unity. (This also corresponds to the theory of a new idealism developed by Bernardo Kastrup, among others, and discussed in more detail in the chapter "The End of the Mechanistic World View".)

The second central law of this world view is *the law of polarity*: All manifest existence is arranged in polarities – day and night, bright and dark, good and evil, life and death, healthy and sick, and so on. It is important to understand that these polarities do not form opposites in the usual sense, which exclude each other, but are rather inseparable sides of a state conditioning each other. Only in the polar form does our world come into existence and differentiations and consciousness become possible. In Absolute Being the opposites collapse, nothing happens, there is no movement and no individuality – it is the source, but no part of the world we know or can know. All mystics point this out: In absolute being there is no cognition, no cogniser, no subject and object. These are all but characteristics of the manifested world, of duality.

More practically speaking, this means that I can always assume that I will find the opposite pole in the vicinity of a strongly pronounced characteristic. Where there is a lot of light, there is also a lot of shadow, folklore correctly says. If a process moves in one direction for a long time, it will for sure come to a turning point and move in the opposite direction; this rule does not only apply to the physical pendulum, but is a cosmic principle, working right into the human psyche and society as well. Every extreme calls for the opposite extreme – this is just as important for health considerations as it is for ethics and politics.

Thirdly, we encounter the *law of the planes* or *levels of existence,* which expresses that – at least in the view of human consciousness – the whole cosmos is arranged in different layers of being. These are on the one hand inseparably connected with each other, but on the other hand they follow their own laws.

Tradition speaks of a hierarchy of existence, which we prefer to express differently today, because the concept of hierarchy, detached from its context and transferred into the political, has had a devastating effect. This very fact is an example of how important it is to understand that the laws of the respective planes of existence must not be interchanged – a mistake that is often made by so-called esoterics.

The *levels* we are talking about here include the following: the physical plane encompasses everything that we can see, touch and measure. This is superimposed and shaped by the etheric or dynamic plane called the life force, Prana or Chi (or Qi). Above it lie the levels of feelings and thoughts, above them again those of the causative will and the pure spirit. In the discussion of homeopathy we will encounter these levels again and enrich them with more content there.

Esoteric schools often set up seven or ten such levels of existence, whereby the number of subdivisions is partly arbitrary, but partly surprisingly consistent in intercultural comparison. Clearly we are dealing here with a universal experience of humanity. An experience that we modern people have largely lost. Contemporary science only deals with the lowest of the levels, the physical one.

64

These levels of existence are by no means presented as abstractions, but experienced in various states of consciousness as very concrete reality, more real than our physical world. According to the hierarchical principle that applies to the planes of existence, the lower planes depend on the higher ones and are therefore in some respects less 'real' for experience. All levels are alive, respectively filled with animated beings. A living being can comprise several levels of existence – such as we humans, who can be physically, dynamically, emotionally, mentally and spiritually present. And a being can be limited to certain levels – angels, for example, we usually do not encounter on the physical level and plants not on the mental one.

The planes of existence penetrate and form each other in a certain order, which leads from the spiritual layers to the more manifested to the material ones. Within this order, an appearance at a certain level is always caused by a higher order. And this 'vertical' causation is regarded as the essential one, which is always superior to the 'horizontal' cause (in the sense of the physical law of causality). It is important to understand this basic principle because many misunderstandings arise from ignorance of it.

An example may illustrate this: We look at an ordinary computer as it stands before us. It consists of many different materials, chips, cables, drives and so on, which are subject to the laws of physics. They form the so-called hardware of the computer. The chips of this hardware must then be programmed with a data language that controls the immediate functions of the machine, the operating system, without which a computer would be nothing but a pile of metal and plastic. The software, i.e. those programmes that interest us as users, can then be turned to the functioning operating system. The laws governing these three levels are not similar to each other. The flip-flop circuits (electronic hardware building blocks of computers) of the chips, on which all computer functions are ultimately based, are determined by the laws of semiconductor physics and electronics. The operating systems have a quite simple grammar for controlling such flip-flop units, which thereby become bits and bytes and so on. The operating system already knows nothing more about the electron currents in silicon. The actual software then is not interested in bits and machine language, but distributes text modules, composes music or creates graphics. The order of these levels is strictly hierarchical and can only be understood from 'top' to 'bottom'. If I wanted to understand the creation of a graphic on the screen solely from the point of view of semiconductor laws, it would be an incomprehensible miracle. Only when I know that there is software with its own graphical laws and a programmer who has put his or her thoughts to the application, does the whole thing make sense.

In a similar situation are those who try to explain the origin of life from the laws of physics and find that the 'accidental' occurrence of complex amino acid structures in the cosmos is extremely unlikely. The same goes for the creation of poems on my screen if I left the chips in the computer to themselves for a thousand years. The laws of life *use* those of physics as the operating system uses the chips and their transistors. And the spiritual laws use those of life just as I can enter my poetic ideas into a word processing program.

This example makes it clear that a hierarchical order of interlocking laws can never be rolled up from 'below'. I cannot derive a poem on the screen from the laws of semiconductor physics, but nevertheless it does not 'contradict' them.

The fourth, the *law of the mandala,* can also be called the *law of symmetrical structures*. We call a mandala a symmetrically divided circular form, sometimes also a square or a hexagon. Symmetry and wholeness are essential to form. All descriptions of the cosmos are arranged in this way.

The simplest basic pattern of this kind is the quaternity of the elements, which are also assigned to the four points of the compass and form circular quarters. Another very typical pattern, the zodiac, shows the symmetry of twelve, which is generally quite common.

The law of the mandala can be seen as an extension of the polarity law. Beyond the formation of polarities and symmetries, it stands above all for the unconditional preservation of wholeness. All structures of the cosmos tend to form completed units or *holons*. In all spontaneous images of the unconscious, in all rituals and myths of mankind, such graphic entities, such mandalas, appear. In the depth psychology of C.G. Jung, the form of the mandala is the pictorial goal of the entire human development process, the individuation, the highest symbol of healing and salvation.

Above all *the law of unity* or *wholeness* prevails and encompasses everything. The Unity of All is the highest of all cosmic principles and the foundation of all others. Everything comes out of the One and everything goes back into it. And only on the basis of this all-embracing Unity can symmetries and analogies be understood meaningfully. The All-Connectedness is a necessary part of the All-Unity.

This unity, too, should not be understood as abstraction, as we find it in philosophy. The unity of the cosmos can be mystically experienced, and the spirit of this unity, often regarded as a deity, carries meaning and intention in itself, is thus intelligent to an extent that far exceeds our understanding.

It is also important that this unity of all being is always understood and experienced as a dynamic one. All being is in motion and filled with the living, dynamic spirit of unity.

There are now attempts to reformulate parts of this explanation of the world with the help of scientific terms. In modern terms, one could understand the microcosm and macrocosm in their unity as parts of a holography: in each fragment, referred to by David Bohm as *holon,* the whole is already completely preserved. This most modern version of the ancient world view described is called *holism.* The biological concept closest to the analogy principle is Rupert Sheldrake's theory of *morphogenetic fields.* Sheldrake's and Bohm's theories, however, lie on the margins of today's mainstream science and are by no means representative of the 'new physics'. Even if they lack the depth and unity of the old view of the world, one feels in them the search for a wholeness of the explanation of the world, which does justice to more than just the mechanistic connections.

It is easy to predict that – as long as humanity survives the next decades as an intact civilisation – a new form of science will also reflect the structures of the old world view in its fundamentals. The search for the *'Theory of Everything'* will find its solution not in a mechanistic formula but in an understanding of the whole that follows the experience of the world as it has always shaped human existence and filled it with meaning.

The Principles of the Hermetic World View

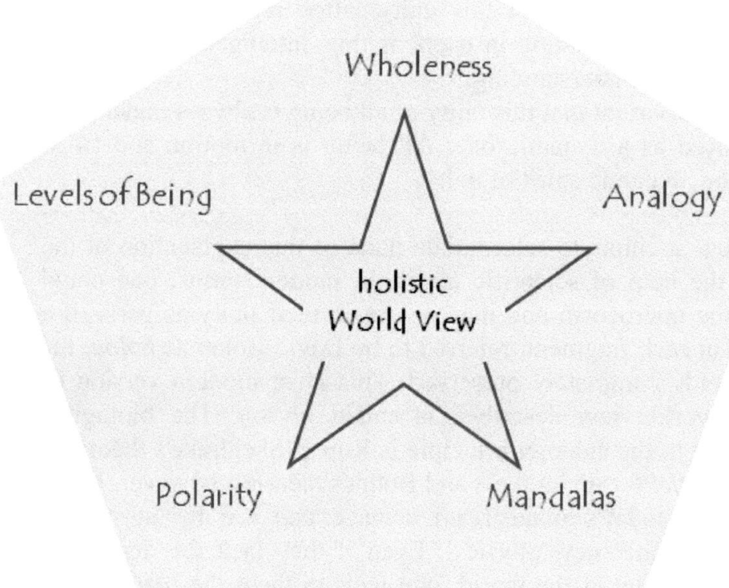

Another Reality II

What kind of 'reality' specifically arises from our imagination according to the laws described so far? What is it like to live in this reality? What distinguishes it from the world view that we are used to? What does it mean when the whole world functions according to the same laws as homeopathy? And what good is it to see the world like this?

The real world[38] is similar to the one we left as children and which we henceforth only encounter in stories. It is a world that we perceive as enchanted, because everything that happens has something to say to us (otherwise it would not happen in our lives). What our life tells us is certainly not always pleasant – especially not when we are ill – yet life always speaks to us. We step out of the apparent meaninglessness of a molecule cluster in an empty universe. The real world is that of spirit and our soul, while the material, visible world is a manifestation of spirit and soul, and is therefore preliminary and changeable.

In contrast to the enchanted world of the child, however, this reality is not based on wishful thinking, but on experience, knowledge and wisdom.

We learn that the processes in our unconscious have much more influence on our health and the course of our destiny than our conscious plans and desires. Our everyday consciousness is only a very small part of our being and has only a moderate influence on our life and our world. Our fate is determined by other forces, which are by no means blind and coincidental, just because they are not subject to our everyday consciousness. In this respect, we are becoming much more modest. For example, we can experience the forces that contribute to our lives in dreams. Or we consciously seek out these deeper layers by means of meditations or imaginary journeys. We may consult a horoscope, the tarot or other interpretive arts to find out about the feelings, forces and developments in our lives that are not accessible to our everyday consciousness.

All events are meaningfully intertwined in the fabric of our life and existence, whether we recognise their meaning immediately or later. Chance as a senseless randomness of events would be an absurd assumption. Likewise our personal life is so closely connected with that of other people and beings that the individualistic concept does not carry us far. There is no individual suffering and no individual redemption – we are all in the same boat. As little as my body is limited when I look closely enough on the physical plane, and as much as I inhale the molecules that the human being next to me has just exhaled, so my personality and soul are not limited and isolated, but part of a comprehensive fabric. And since all this has a meaning, also the plans and wishes of my everyday consciousness are integrated into a much larger context, which for my small overview is not strategised and not comprehensible.

We experience many qualities of the other world view when we are seriously ill: our relationships carry us and become important; our achievements count for little, and our money has limited value. A hopeful gesture weighs more than all statistics. The warmth of a hand makes us more comfortable than tubes and pills. Such perceptions are not 'subjective' and 'incidental', but they show us the real world. In severe illness we wake up from the nightmare of machines, money, cars and power, of performance, pressure, speed, precision, time and files. We wake up in a world that consists of people, bodies and emotions that is warm and changeable, painful perhaps, but alive and meaningful. We feel what is important to us and what is unimportant to us, who we like to have around us and who we don't.

The wisdom of personal experiences counts more than learned knowledge, trust weighs more than external power, authentic feelings tell us deeper truths about the world than theories, the sense for the course of our destiny takes us further than our conscious plans, the conceptual content of our words is not as important as the forces resonating in them, and how we act in our dreams can be more important than the activities during the day. – Our culture, our schools and our education prepare us badly for the real reality. That is why many people shy away from it and prefer to remain in the relative trance state of our everyday life. This makes our culture as a whole inflexible and narrow and leads to the fact that we are not up to the demands of reality and thereby hurt the fabric of life.

The expansion of consciousness from the everyday trance to a greater reality often happens through unsettling experiences, whereby

70

serious illnesses are probably the most frequent. Near-death experiences, deaths of relatives, drug experiences, spontaneous spiritual experiences, encounters with other cultures or internal crises can provide other wake-up calls. No matter which way we come, finally we all open ourselves to the same reality. Thus a serious illness and the contact with a holistic healing can change us forever.

Homeopathy and its Spiritual Roots in Hermeticism

Homeopathy seems to fit seamlessly into the holistic view of reality described above. The basic laws of hermeticism, the 'eternal philosophy' or alchemy are summarised above as the *law of analogy*, the *law of polarity*, the *law of the levels of being*, the *law of the mandala* and the *law of unity*. In terms of homeopathy, it looks like this:

1) The homeopathic *law of similarity* is nothing more than a specialised version of the universal law of analogy, correspondence or resonance.[39] It is interesting to note that Hahnemann – unlike the people of ancient times – has collected, arranged and written down a vast amount of precise observations to confirm the law of analogy or simile. By this he already proved to be a man of modernity and an important forerunner of scientific medicine.

2) The *law of polarities* is manifested in homeopathy in the form of primary and secondary reactions to the intake of remedies, which run exactly opposite to each other and appear in prescription practice as initial reactions, suppression, etc. This basic principle of polarity can also be found in many remedy images by showing a number of exactly opposite properties.

3) The view that the world contains different *planes of existence* that penetrate and influence each other is the basis of all Hahnemann's thoughts. Let us take an exemplary sentence from the Organon (§9): *"In the healthy state of the human being, the spiritual vital force (autocracy), which as dynamis invigorates the material body*

(organism), prevails unrestrictedly and keeps all its parts in admirably harmonious course of life, in feelings and activities, so that our inherent, rational spirit can freely use this living, healthy tool for the higher purpose of our existence".

Here we see the human being consisting of the material body, which – as long as it lives – is animated by the dynamis, so that both can be tools of the spirit, which in turn is subject to a higher purpose. It was never in Hahnemann's interest to formulate philosophical aspects in more detail; neither did he give them any quasi-religious interpretations. He was a physician only and not an esoteric, but he leaves no doubt about his view of the world and of the human constitution.

In explaining the principle of potentisation, we also encounter the necessity of being able to separate the essence of a substance from its materiality. Hahnemann points this out again and again and with this intention – to separate the essence or spirit and the material substance in the laboratory – clearly places himself in the tradition of alchemy, even though the process he uses seems to be new. The potentisation with alternating dilution and shaking (*succussion*) corresponds to the alchemical 'raising' of a substance by alternating distillation and condensation. And when we read in Hahnemann's book how the process of potentising makes the actual essence of a medicine stand out from the material and become clearer, this is almost inevitably reminiscent of the alchemical descriptions of the maturation of matter by alchemical art: *"This makes it extremely probable that matter by means of such dynamisation (development of its true, inner, medicinal being) will dissolve completely into its individual spiritual being in the end and can therefore be regarded in its raw state, actually only as consisting of this undeveloped, spirit-like being." (Hahnemann, Organon, §270, Note 7)* And *"Medicinal substances are not dead substances in the ordinary sense; rather their true essence is merely dynamic spiritual – is pure energy ...". (Hahnemann, Materia Medica Pura, Part 6, p.11)*

Hahnemann understood the nature of the disease as non-material, as a force (he called it 'potency') which was present at the level of the life force, the dynamis. Several times he emphasised that nothing of it could be found in the physical, material body and that it was subject to completely different laws. So it has a clear logic that even the remedy cannot start at the material level. Disease potency and remedy potency encounter each other at the same level, which Hahnemann calls partly dynamic, partly essential or spiritual. From this context it follows that humans as well as nature as a whole must be assigned a level of existence that is not material in its essence. From this level the essential life impulses emanate, as well as disease and healing. The material plane is only the sphere of effect, an outer mirror of the actually invisible event. Such a concept has no place and no meaning in scientific thought and theories. Which does not mean that there is a contradiction between both views. They just focus on different levels of being and different methods of describing them.

There have been a number of attempts to translate the homeopathic theses into cybernetic self-regulation or into system-theoretical terms. But in such a process, fundamental factors of the concept are always lost. Hahnemann said very clearly what he meant. And we, too, can understand his thoughts and research well if we apply a suitable world view and do not try to somehow bend homeopathy into our accustomed thinking.[40]

between homeopathy and alchemy, respectively hermeticism

The question arises why such an obvious connection between the homeopathic doctrine and the hermetic tradition, as it has been demonstrated here, does not seem to have played a major role in the history of homeopathy.

Homeopathy originated in the Age of Enlightenment, when most of human knowledge and ancient traditions fell into suppression and oblivion. In almost all branches of human knowledge, it progressed as if there had been no serious transmission of knowledge before. With the pathos of pure observation and experience, it was overlooked that every observation is theory-driven and that every theory follows certain cognitive interests. In that era people believed they could reinvent the wheel and looked down on the world views of our ancestors with a patronising expression. Only with the help of the suppression of all historical and philosophical connections was it possible in such an ideological climate to save hermetic ideas into the incipient modern age.[41]

Nevertheless, there were provable historical links. We know[42] that Hahnemann, through his extensive reading, had made enough acquaintance with alchemical and hermetic world interpretations to know of their basic principles and to know their procedures. During his stay in Sibiu in Transylvania in 1779, Hahnemann had contact with alchemical literature during the inventory of Baron Brukenthal's library, for example the *Medicina Spagyrica* by Rhumelius[43], where he expressly advocated a treatment according to the principle 'similia similibus curentur'. In addition, Hahnemann was a Freemason and in this way also had access to the hermetic tradition, which – partly referred to as Rosicrucian knowledge – was still passed on in Masonic lodges.

Officially, Hahnemann always distanced himself from these traditions. He remained an outspoken representative of the ideals of the Enlightenment, although he lived simultaneously with the Romantics and Goethe, who had already embarked on new (and old) paths. If Hahnemann adopted or further developed hermetic knowledge, then he was either not aware of it or intentionally concealed it in order not to expose his teaching to increased criticism. Since he did not shun the confrontation with his contemporaries anywhere else, the latter is rather unlikely. So we can assume that via Hahnemann there was only an intellectual approach to the thinking style of hermeticism.

However, there has been an important direct link between Kent and Swedenborg. James Tyler Kent (1849 – 1916) can probably be regarded as one of the most influential homeopaths after Hahnemann. He is the author of the most important repertory of homeopathic remedies, as well as of the most frequently used series of potencies in the prescriptions: C 30, C 200, C 1000, C 10000, and of still current authoritative works on materia medica and homeopathic philosophy. Like many other important North American homeopaths of his time, Kent was a follower of the Swedish mystic, visionary and Christian esoteric Emanuel Swedenborg. Here the closeness of the homeopathic method to an esoteric world view was most evident. The ease with which Kent was able to explain homeopathy within this framework made his philosophical lectures on The Organon the most important theoretical source for subsequent homeopaths – albeit neglecting the spiritual basis Kent himself had for it. With his concept of the 'simple substance'[44] for Hahnemann's *dynamis*, Kent again approaches the alchemical idea of a Materia prima, right up to the building of terms. In his explanations of their effect and position in the organism, he formulates a comprehensive esoteric theory of life force far beyond Hahnemann's concept.

Last but not least, since Hahnemann's time all esoteric currents of the Occident have recognised and used homeopathy as a related method. The best-known example is Rudolf Steiner's anthroposophy, whose medicine also works with potentiated substances and whose physicians partly also resort to classical homeopathy. On the other hand, the repeatedly asserted rejection of the use of high potencies by Steiner is based on a rumour. There is no verifiable statement by Steiner in this direction. On the contrary, like other esoterics, he has advocated homeopathy. However, medicine on the basis of the anthroposophical conception of humans is an independent method with its own therapeutic principles and remedies.

4) The *law of the mandala* or of symmetrically structured wholes (*holons*) is the one that is least implemented in homeopathy as yet. Hahnemann's long refusal to speculate or to formulate comprehensive theories led to the fact that he collected and documented an immense abundance of analogies between humans, characters, diseases and natural substances, but was never able to apply a meaningful order to them. It was only at an advanced age that he made an attempt with his miasm theory to assume three basic diseases, the so-called 'miasms' Psora, Sycosis and Syphilis, for human disease symptoms as well as for homeopathic remedies.

Later generations of homeopaths have not stopped discussing this problem and inventing new systems of order. They joined Hahnemann's three miasms with the tuberculinic one as the fourth, in which we then easily recognise the four elements fire (syphilis), air (tuberculosis), water (sycosis) and earth (psora); or they used the periodic system of the chemical elements as an ordering principle, or the natural kingdoms of minerals, plants and animals. None of these orders has been able to assert itself so far, and the problem has yet to be solved by another generation of homeopaths.

The reason for this scepticism of Hahnemann and many of his successors regarding analogue systems of order was based on the fact that at his time the handling of the principles of analogy in the form of the theory of signatures and the widespread humoralism (the doctrine of temperaments and humours [liquids of the body]) was very outmoded[45] and was practised only as a semi-understood or misunderstood relic on the basis of ancient writings – much to the disadvantage of the patients, as Hahnemann repeatedly had to find out. He then rejected not only the abuse but also the method itself. During his lifetime, he no longer came to the conclusion that he had probably thrown out the baby with the bath water here. With the miasm theory he tried to regain in a speculative way what he had lost from tradition, but the attempt became stuck right at the beginning.

It proves to be advantageous here to refer a method (homeopathy) to a more comprehensive system (the hermetic world view) in order to discover and clear structural gaps in the method. The holistic systems of understanding the world carry completeness in themselves, since they always represent divisions of the unity.

76

5) The *wholeness* and *unity of being* in a universal consciousness is the general basic principle of all complete and comprehensive human world views, however they present themselves in detail.

The will to refer to this unity occurs in homeopathy as the *law of intention*, of directed will, in which all other factors are gathered and given their meaning. Without a clear intention of healing as a connection with the "higher purpose of our existence" (as Hahnemann called it), there can be no holistic healing. This is never conceivable as a forced automatic, but only as an art, as the ever unique act of reconnection to the whole.

The Principles of Homeopathy
and the World view on which they are based

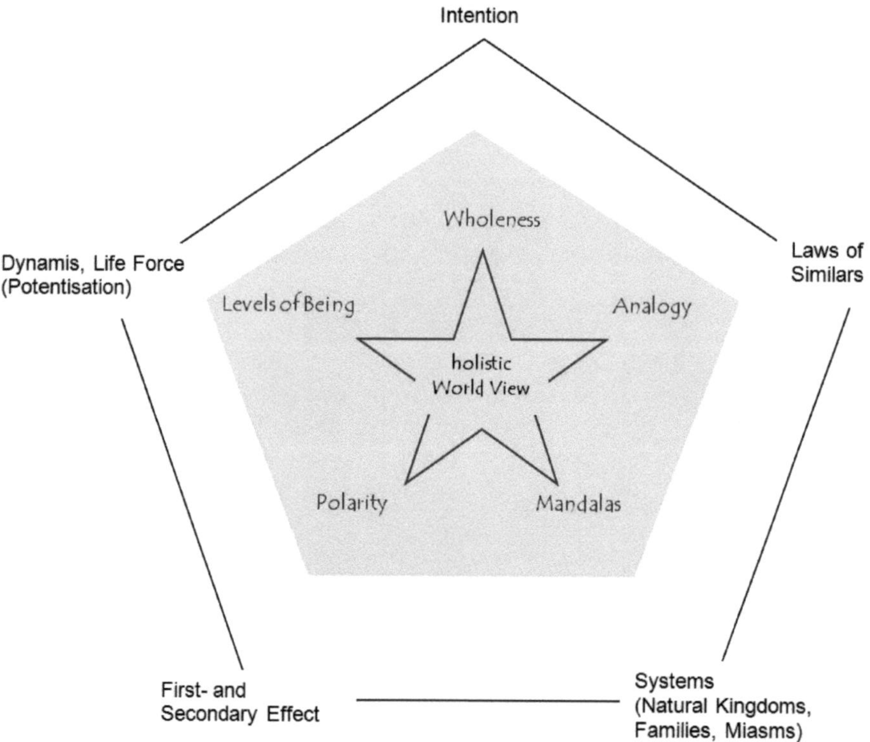

Principles of homeopathy and their roots in the ⇒	holistic/ magical / hermetic world view
- the law of similarity "Similia similibus curentur"	1) analogy: "As above so below" – the law of correspondence and resonance in the micro- and macrocosmos
- the law of first and after-effects (the basis of the medicinal effect according to Hahnemann)	2) polarity: nothing exists without the effect of its opposite
- the action of the life force, *dynamis*, unlike the physical body, which is called a tool of the spirit. (The possibility of potentisation is based on the possibility of separating these levels from each other.)	3) hierarchy of the levels of being: Besides the physical level there is the level of the life force, the level of the psyche, the rational mind and the level of the spirit – in the microcosm as well as the macrocosm.
- systems of order or relations, miasms and nature kingdoms	4) mandalas – structured entities: each whole (*holon*) is symmetrically structured in itself
- the intention: to connect us in healing with the "higher purpose of our existence"	5) unity: on the highest level of existence everything is one, connected, in relationship and animated.

To express again what has been said in a different way: The effect of a homeopathic remedy is based on the fact that there are universal patterns in nature, whether you call them archetypes, ideas, morphogenetic fields, spirits or whatever. These patterns determine all events on all levels. The spiritual patterns can be manifested as external substances or represented in such substances – that is the concern of alchemy as well as of homeopathic remedy preparation. The task of homeopathic treatment is to find this pattern in its disease-causing form, to name it and to provide an encounter with the same principle in the form of a medicine.

In ancient times, illness was often described as an evil spirit having control over a person's condition. Healing was based on recognising and naming this spirit. If you only knew the name of a spirit, then it had lost its power – in modern language: if you can identify and name the offending pattern, you can provide healing.

Depth psychology and astrology work according to the same principle. Depth-psychological work includes the recognition of basic archetypal patterns in people's behaviour, fantasies and dreams, their becoming aware and further developing into patterns that express a wholeness. These archetypal patterns can be found in the individual psyche as well as in the collective, i.e. in cultural testimonies. Astrology names the patterns of behaviour and perception of human beings with the help of the traditional symbols of the zodiac and planets. Healing and mental development take place through recognition of these complex symbolic patterns. Holistic body therapies, such as craniosacral therapy, osteopathy or bioenergetic methods, seek the mental patterns mainly in their physical expression and release them on this level. This often sets free associated feelings, images or memories, but the focus is not on mental processing.

What is special about the homeopathic approach is the consistent inclusion of the physical and mental levels: "Body and mind are like two different, but interrelated, complementary stages on which the same directional force, individuality, performs the same piece, only in two different languages, so to speak".[46] In homeopathy, it is necessary to reconcile these two languages and to understand their common pattern.

For some, the question whether homeopathy can be applied by Christian believers may seem strange as such. But in certain (evangelical) Christian circles there are obviously problems with homeopathy as well as with other holistic healing methods. These are considered 'occult' or 'esoteric' and therefore reprehensible.

A few clarifying thoughts: in the ancient world view and until modern times, a general distinction was made between white and black magic. If one wants to use this distinction at all, and black magic doesn't always mean the magic of the others, the following would be an understanding of it: magic is any form of influence on the outer world or the psyche of other people that transcends everyday events. White magic was one that was embedded in the respective accepted spiritual context, i.e. had a spiritual connection and saw itself in the service of the whole. Black magic was the manipulation of the world for one's own benefit and without considering the community and the whole. According to the traditional world view (and the Christian positions mentioned are within the framework of this ancient concept of good and evil[47]), the modern materialistic sciences clearly represent a form of black magic: They manipulate the world without having a spiritual connection and intention. So anyone who, from a Christian point of view, rejects the influence of homeopathic remedies on health, because this is usually not done with reference to the Christian deity, would all the more have to reject any scientifically based method of healing. After all, homeopathy still sees itself as holistic, and Hahnemann even referred to an idea of God that is quite close to the Christian one, and placed his homeopathy at His service. In contrast, orthodox medicine is decidedly godless.

We know from the Bible that Jesus explicitly gave his followers the mandate to heal and cast out spirits. He certainly didn't have chemotherapy in mind. The way Jesus (and other healers of his time and tradition) dealt with sufferers has much in common with the homeopathic mindset.

Hahnemann himself was a very devout man, whose image of God was strongly influenced by Christianity. As a Freemason, he had freed himself from confessional restrictions. It was typical for him, for example, that he spoke of the "approach to the spirit worshipped by the inhabitants of all solar systems".[48]

Therapeutic work in the context described here, requires a rethinking of the applied concepts and the development of a (for us) new trust in these laws. Thinking in mechanistic categories and factual constraints, in orthodox medical disease concepts and processes, in theories of pathogens and infections, of chemistry and substance has become so much part of our flesh and blood that it can take a long time before we can really get involved in a holistic conception of the world and therapy.

The most important principle here is that we follow the order of the planes of existence and assume that the material structure always follows the flow of energy. The life energy is not something that flows in the material body like blood or lymph; rather, it is the formative mental structure in which matter is embedded. As Meister Eckhart said, it is not that the soul is in the body, but the body in the soul. Here are a few quotes from Kent, probably the most authoritative homeopath after Hahnemann:

"Each and everything that appears before the eyes is but the representative of its cause, and there is no cause except in the interior. Cause does not flow from the outermost of man to the interior, because man is protected against such a state of affairs. Causes exist in such subtle form that they cannot be seen by the eye. There is no disease that exists of which the cause is known to man by the eye or by the microscope. Causes are infinitely too fine to be observed by any instrument of precision. They are so immaterial that they correspond to and operate upon the interior nature of man, and they are ultimated in the body in the form of tissue changes that are recognized by the eye. Such tissue changes must be understood as the results of disease only or the physician will never perceive what disease cause is, what disease is, what potentization is, or what the nature of life is. This is what Hahnemann meant when he speaks of the fundamental causes as existing in chronic miasm." (Kent, Lectures on Homeopathic Philosophy, p.50)
"Allopaths are really taking the sequence for the consequence, thus leading to a false theory, the bacteria theory. You may destroy the bacteria and yet not destroy the disease. The susceptibility remains the

82

same, and only those that are susceptible will take the disease. Bacteria have a use, for there is nothing in the whole world that does not have a use, and there is nothing sent on earth to destroy man. The bacteria theory would make it appear that the all-wise Creator has sent these micro-organisms here to make man sick. We see from this paragraph that Hahnemann did not adopt any such theory as bacteriology." (Kent p.52)
"All the imitations of miasms are found in drugs. There is no miasm of the human race that does not have its imitation in drugs. The animal kingdom has in itself the image of sickness, and the vegetable and mineral kingdoms in like manner, and if man were perfectly conversant with the substances of these three kingdoms he could treat the whole human race. By application the physician must fill his mind with images that correspond to the sicknesses of the human race." (Kent, p.46)

What else does the recognition of the hermetic world view mean in therapeutic work? For example, the polarity: Every life situation represents a whole, and I can always assume that there is an antithesis to everything I directly perceive that belongs to the truth of the whole. If, for example, a patient experiences his relationship exclusively as a victim, then the counterforce, the perpetratorship, will also emerge in the course of the therapy. If someone seems very depressed, I can expect a phase of violent aggression during the healing process, and so on. If I am aware of this, then I know that as a therapist I do not have to bring about any of this. The therapeutic process lives from this natural regularity, and I can accompany this and make it conscious.

Another point is the handling of homeopathic remedies, globules. If I imagine a homeopathic remedy in principle as a medicine, then there are many paradoxes and problems, not only with the high dilution. For example, in the course of each homeopathic potentisation, the alternating rubbing, diluting and shaking of a certain starting substance in lactose and alcohol-water mixture, countless impurities of the devices, the starting substance, the laboratory air, the laboratory technician's breathing air and the solvents are shaken and further potentiated even under the greatest care and highest cleanliness of the laboratory. And even if we do not take this into consideration, the lactose is always potentiated as well with every potentisation and must have left its traces in every known remedy picture. – How does homeopathic potency 'know' which of the many substances in the triturated and succussed mixture it depends on? How can the original 'sound' still be distinguished from the 'noise' that has been amplified with potency heights that lie beyond the material? There are no meaningful explanations for this in mechanistic thinking. We must dare the spiritual leap and explain the effects with the main principle of magic: Intention is (almost) everything! A remedy becomes what the manufacturer *wants* and *imagines*. Consequently this takes us to the inseparable combination of laboratory work and soul work, of (al)chemical knowledge and trained willpower and imagination, which is typical for alchemical work. The art of alchemy as well as of homeopathy is now to master the balancing act between the inner process and the technical skill. Both aspects are equally necessary; neither can be overridden by the other. Homeopathy, too, cannot be accomplished either by computer alone or by intuition alone. The ideal case is when the tools of the trade are mastered so confidently that the attention can be completely free for the movements in mind and spirit.

Perhaps the most important insight from the hermetic world view for the treatment is that we as therapists always sit in the same boat with the patients. The often-perceived haughtiness of doctors in regard to their patients or the psychoanalytic 'abstinence' as attempts to take objective positions towards other people, are illusionary and must fail. All those involved in a system such as a family, a working group, a therapy situation are always closely intertwined on many levels and share the same dynamic, mirroring each other. Many therapists are aware of the phenomenon that during their own crises many patients come with similar problems. Here, too, the popular wisdom applies that the same joins the same, and opposites attract each other, which means for us homeopaths: Similia similibus curentur.

"The alchemists looked for the meaning, for the causes of the phenomena. The materialistic sciences are satisfied with the description of the facts. They are explanatory sciences, not understanding sciences."[49]

"As little as the astrology of the past can be described as the precursor of today's astronomy, as little can the alchemy of many thousands of years be regarded as the precursor of modern chemistry, around one hundred and fifty years old. (...) So it should be pointed out here once again that this is not at all about the correctness or incorrectness of this or that seemingly incisive astronomical, chemical or physical fact, but about fundamentally having a different orientation in the sense of a dynamic-spiritual world view in contrast to the sciences of the present, still spiritually alienated despite quantum mechanics and relativity theory."[50]

Materialistic Science and Homeopathy

The question remains as to what relationship such an alchemistically and hermetically determined homeopathy can have to the currently established materialistic science.

The relationship between homeopathy and science as a whole is difficult to determine because the word 'science' usually refers to only a certain, historically recent and short-lived form of human knowledge. In principle, homeopathy fulfils all the criteria of science: it observes systematically; it processes all the accumulated knowledge and continually compares it with older data; it constantly compares and systematises the results of the work of all those involved and constantly checks them against new observations; it is subject to constant self-criticism and self-control through the practical application of the results and also through the international exchange of researching and applying homeopaths. But it does not fit into the system of the current mechanistic sciences because it cannot be derived from their assumptions about the world. It is part of a different kind of science with different prerequisites and different approaches. Different world views, however, produce different sciences that describe the world – correctly – yet in different ways. This has already been described in detail in the chapter on paradigms.

A common cliché has it that homeopathic effects would contradict modern scientific laws – for example, by the height of the potentisations, the famous drop into Lake Constance. However, this is not the case and is based on a fundamental misunderstanding of what constitutes the materialistic sciences. A fact or observation can never contradict a science from the outset, because it is the objective of sciences to explain the observed reality, but not to determine what can and cannot be real. Brecht gives us a very nice example of a false understanding of science in his drama about Galilei (4th picture). Galileo invites the scholars to look through his telescope and convince themselves of the existence of the Jupiter moons. They refuse with the argument that the known model of the world declares the moons' existence impossible.

Similarly, in the name of science[51] today, there are arguments against homeopathy or other phenomena that cannot be explained mechanistically (see chapter "Homeopathy and its opponents"). In fact, current mechanistic science cannot satisfactorily explain the observations and procedures of the homeopathic method. But in this there is no contradiction and no problem in materialistic science or in homeopathy. Contrary to metaphysical assumptions, a scientific theory can in principle not refer to the whole world, but only to a clearly limited area of its research. Outside this scope of valid research and theory, statements of the science concerned are pointless. We don't usually learn where these boundaries lie as there is an unspoken conviction that they could be postponed indefinitely until orthodox science can explain everything.

This belief that reality is limited to the results of contemporary materialistic science and its theories is not a scientific attitude, but a kind of ideological fundamentalism called *scientism*. On the part of the opponents of homeopathy, a kind of scientism of this kind is usually put forward, which refers to the reality model of physics before relativity and quantum theory. This model (more or less of the end of the 19th century), with its absolutism of objectivity, determinism and strict causality, has not been cherished in the circles of real scientists since the first half of the last century, but apparently still haunts many people's minds and, in the absence of real scientific relevance, has solidified into a mechanistic belief system which is put forward with the vehemence of fundamentalist conviction. In this respect, it is important in discussions to distinguish between science and *scientism*, a belief in a certain past phase of scientific knowledge, since the two have little to do with each other.

Within their respective fields of application, the statements of our modern materialistic sciences are of course correct and valuable; and no homeopath could contradict them on the basis of his or her experience. However, the homeopathic context does not lie within the area of their competence and can therefore not contradict the orthodox mechanistic science. There is no contradiction here, but two fundamentally different approaches in different levels of existence.

Healing is related to the function of certain tissues in the same way as love is to certain hormonal fluctuations. Although I can state that healing, as well as love, has typical physical side effects, neither healing nor love can be explained by these physical side effects. In this respect, healing in its verifiability and scientific explication can be compared well with love. It is a well-known phenomenon the nature of which cannot be understood scientifically. And even love cannot be reproduced under laboratory conditions or in double-blind studies. But no one would doubt that it exists. **Love, destiny, healing, life and death will always remain phenomena which, in their essence, elude scientific access.**

"Since this natural healing law is authenticated in all pure experiments and all genuine experiences of the world, the fact therefore exists. So little depends on the scientific explanation, how this happens, and I set little value on trying the like. But the following view proves to be the most probable, since [it] is based on a lot of experiential premises."
(§28 – Organon)

Homeopathy does not treat with verbal explanations or purely mental influences, but with so-called remedies, i.e. material carriers. Of course, this always raises the question of what happens physically or chemically when such remedies are administered. In the high potencies of homeopathic remedies there is no chemically detectable starting substance. Therefore we see a number of studies and considerations about the effects of trituration, dilution and succussion.

The physically best-elaborated models are those that try to explain the transmission of homeopathic information through a 'memory of water'. Water molecules are supposed to have the natural ability to form molecule clusters which are very complex and highly differentiated (similar to snow crystals) and which are physically long lasting[52]. Like an information matrix, these could multiply and differentiate themselves through rhythmic shaking in the solution. Like water, lactose and alcohol are strongly dipolar molecules that could have similar properties.

Yet even in scientifically well-informed and precise works, such as those by Resch and Gutmann, there are only physical models that *could be* suitable as the material basis of homeopathy. But already

88

within physics such models have hypothetical character and move at the edge or beyond the edge of the present state of knowledge. Whether homeopathic laws will be able to follow these models, if more is known about them, remains open and speculative.

In accordance with our physical thinking habits, physical metaphors were formed in the twentieth century to help explain all possible non-physical connections. Thus, psychic phenomena (telepathy, haunting, etc.) were explained with the help of so-called 'Psi' energies, waves or neutrino currents. The different qualities of the ground and in the landscape were called earth 'radiation' or 'grids of ley lines'. The formation of metaphors to interpret the new and the foreign with the help of known structures is common and legitimate. We just have to avoid confusing such metaphor with scientific statements. The 'energies', 'vibrations' or 'resonances' which we are talking about in this context have nothing to do with the physical concept of energy. This is a quantity within a system of mathematical formulae, and quantifiability is as much a part of the essence of this concept as are unambiguous units of measurement. Metaphors, of course, do not provide this. They can have a descriptive value, but have nothing to do with scientific considerations.

Apart from the lack of a physical basis, the concept of energy implies much that cannot be found in homeopathic application (see also the chapter "Dynamis – the life force"). For example, more energy would also have to produce more effect and thus the effect of a remedy would depend strongly on the number of globules taken, which is not the case. A C30 would then have to be ten times weaker or stronger than a C3, which is also not the case. If we really want to use a physical metaphor, then that of the field would be closer (although here, too, the field strength and the vector character of a field cannot be classified in a meaningful way).

It is better to drop the misleading and clumsy pseudo-physical concepts and – like Hahnemann – talk about the spirit or essence of a remedy. It may one day be possible to prove the physical way in which the structure of the starting substances is passed on in the carriers (water, alcohol, lactose). That would certainly be fascinating, but remains open for the time being.

In recent decades, a number of efforts have been made to research the effects of homeopathic therapy on a scientific basis, i.e. to apply the same criteria to it as to other forms of medicine.[53] This was done under three questions: On the one hand, a) an attempt was made to clarify by means of controlled clinical studies, double-blind, whether homeopathic remedies have any effect at all that can be distinguished from placebo effects. Secondly, b) physical and biochemical experiments were carried out in order to get closer to a scientific understanding of the mechanisms of action of high potencies. And c), there were general outcome studies to find out the effectiveness of homeopathic therapy regardless of its possible mechanisms, but just having in mind the well-being of the patients.

a) Is homeopathy effective at all? In spite of the difficulty of applying an unfamiliar testing method to homeopathy that does not take into account the holistic nature of the method, and in spite of the considerable methodological problems that are raised anyway by double-blind studies and the unclear concept of placebo[54], the effectiveness studies on homeopathic medicines have turned out to be so favourable in sum that even a group of critics describes the arguments of homeopathic therapists as "an enviable position".[55] This means that even under the most unfavourable conditions and with an often irrelevant study design[56] it could be demonstrated that homeopathic remedies have a different effect than placebo.

b) Are highly potentiated substances physically present and can they be observed by measurements? The basic investigations on the physical and biochemical behaviour of high potencies seem to have at least provided evidence that potentiated substances behave differently than non-potentiated substances of the same dilution level. Similar investigations and proofs have long been provided by anthroposophical scientists who, by means of qualitative detection methods (e.g. drop images, thin-layer chromatography), have shown that biodynamically grown plants can be distinguished from conventional plants – and in this sense, methods of biodynamic farming (e.g. 'rhythmisation") as well as potentisation are alchemical methods which are not expected to show any differences from a superficial chemical point of view.

Ironically, clinical studies on homeopathic therapy are often subject to much stricter scientific standards than orthodox medicine in order not to be disqualified by formal errors or statistical weaknesses.[57]

c) Studies that focus not on the evidence but on the effectiveness of homeopathic treatment in the outcome just compare different ways of treating certain groups of patients and look at the outcome in terms of health, happiness of the patients and economic viability. Such studies have been done especially by health insurances and on a large scale in Switzerland[58], where the result was to legally settle homeopathy and other CAM methods in the national health care, because they were scientifically clearly proven to be effective, helpful and inexpensive.

In summary, it can be said that to date scientific research has shown that homeopathic effects are at least clearly existent in the horizon of a mechanistic perception and interpretation of the world. If we sufficiently refine the measurement procedures, the presence of such effects can be observed. Similar to parapsychological research, however, the possible statements do not go beyond the identification of the mere existence of such effects, which form anomalies within mechanistic theory. How they actually come about, what their inner laws are, and all the questions that concern us homeopaths in our daily practice remain unexplained and unaffected. That is the current state of affairs, and given our fundamental reflections on these issues, I would not expect anything to change significantly.[59]

A decisive point in the debate on scientific methodology is that a holistic approach needs a different scientific framework from a mechanistic one. Such a different approach is based on the basic assumption that a whole can*not* be meaningfully understood in terms of components. A future science of nature will certainly develop its own criteria for this.

Another interesting connection between homeopathy and modern materialistic science is that homeopathy can be regarded as a precursor of modern scientific methods within medicine. This refers to the method to learn by means of precise observation of the sick person.

Although Paracelsus had already made observations at the bedside – as homeopaths love to call it – he was so far ahead of his time that no direct imitators could be found. It was not until Hahnemann's time that concrete observations in clinical practice as well as experimental findings (the remedy provings on healthy people) were systematically combined and laws derived from them. This complies with the ideal of an inductively proceeding science and the theoretical basis of today's mechanistic orthodox medicine.

Within scientific medicine, Samuel Hahnemann is indeed one of the pioneers of experimental and systematically observational methodology.[60] To be fair, however, it must be said that in doing so – in Paracelsian tradition – he only helped to overcome a tragic low of European science. In the Arab world there had been better medicine for a long time, and before academic medicine there had always been a wealth of healing methods among the people in Europe, too, which – apart from certain superstitious elements – were based on concrete experiences of many centuries. In the following chapter we would like to connect to these old and ancient traditions. Here, too, modern homeopathy picks up on mankind's oldest body of knowledge.

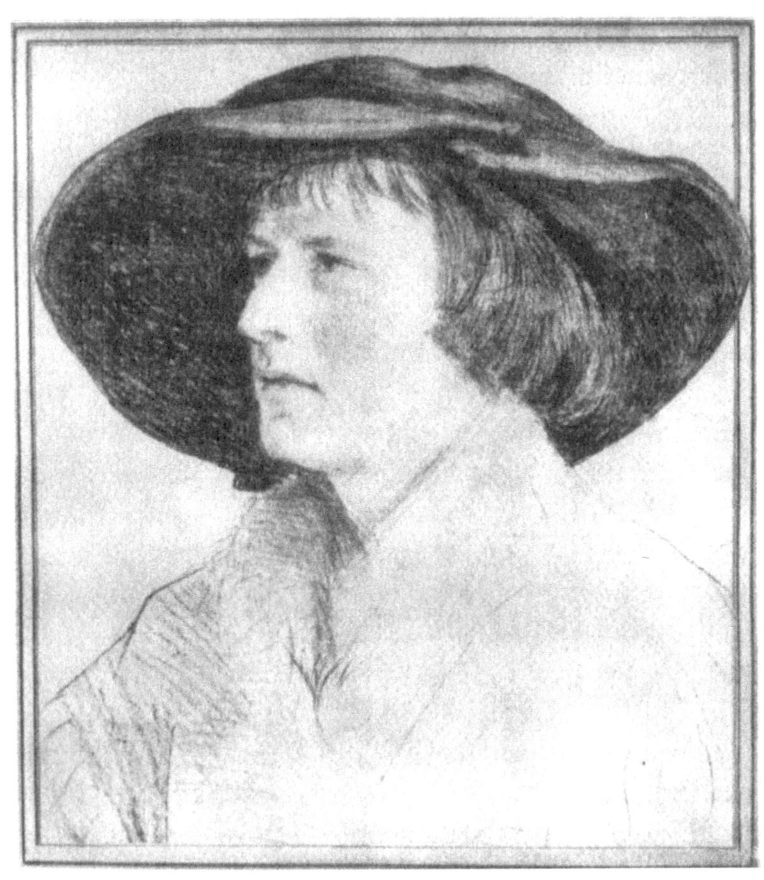

Theophrastus Bombastus of Hohenheim (born 1493, canton Schwyz, died 1541 in Salzburg (drawing by Hans Holbein the Younger, 16th century)

I can lose my eyes and still live.
I can lose my hands and still live.
I can lose my legs and still live.
I can lose my ears, nose, hair, and still live.

But if I lose the earth, I die.
  If I lose the water, I die.
    If I lose the air, I die.
      If I lose the sun, I die.
        If I lose the plants, animals, stars, I die.

          What is my true body?

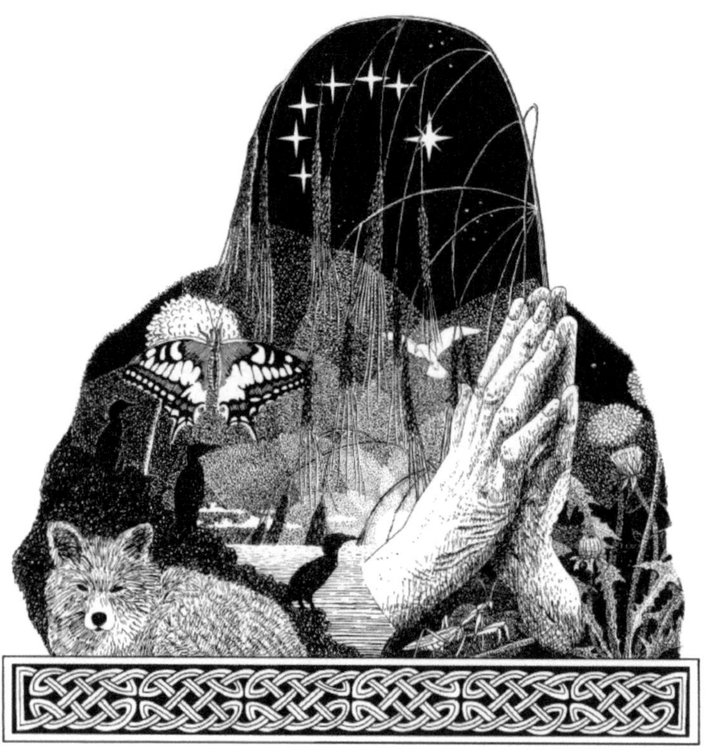

94

Medicine Men and Women of Today

Shamanism is much older than alchemy and goes back to the beginnings of human history. Many see in shamanism the origin of all religion and all healing, the shaman being the archetype and precursor of the priest, the magician, the physician, the healer and the saint. Or rather, we should imagine the shaman to be female in origin, especially when it comes to times so far back in history. As the healers and priestesses of the rural population, the so-called witches were the shamans of Europe until modern times. Paracelsus, the great healer in the dawn of modern times and father of empirical medicine, said he had all his knowledge of wise women. In this respect, through Paracelsus and Hahnemann there is a recognisable spiritual line back to the early history of healing.

However, the connection between homeopathy and shamanism should not be made here in a speculative historical sense. Rather, it is a matter of considering the role of the healers in different cultural contexts. In many peoples there was for a long time a coexistence of shamanism and priesthood. The priesthood represented rather a formal, static aspect of religion, while the shamans could give access to the spiritual realm from very personal experiences. Often conflicts or at least a certain polarity arose as a result. Shamans who could heal and perform magic and had access to unpredictable powers were visited, but remained eerie, incalculable.

European history of the last centuries was overwhelmingly monopolised by the priesthood, and not only in the church-religious sense. Due to the witch burnings of the early modern period and the Renaissance (C 16th–17th), the competitors of the newly establishing medical profession, disappeared. At the same time the modern sciences emerged, and in philosophy the Enlightenment cleared away traditional metaphysics. The mass exterminations of witches, midwives, healers and many other people organised by the state and the churches are often transferred to the dark Middle Ages. However, the mass murders took place during the times of Reformation, Renaissance, Enlightenment and developing sciences. When everything 'shamanic' had disappeared from European culture for a long time, the 'disenchantment' of the world was thought to have succeeded. Small counter-cultural movements such as Romanticism, Spiritism, Art Nouveau or early youth movements and the like remained marginal, but were sufficient to preserve certain basic philosophical ideas and also the remains of another medicine.

Conventional medicine today plays the social role of the established priesthoods, while the different forms of holistic medicine play the role of the shamans, simultaneously needed and suspected. In the well-known role clichés of the heroic physician and the quack doctor or miracle worker this relationship is clearly displayed[62]. In this respect it seems justified to speak of the 'medicine men and women of today' and to describe by them a social role and form of healing that has existed since time immemorial, since humans have existed. In our time religion plays an ever-smaller role in public, but individual health has risen to a quasi-religious significance that tips the scale of values of most people. The conflict of role between the medical establishment as priesthood and the alternative healers as 'witches', which is indicated here, gains a socially influential role. – This division of roles raises the question of whether it really makes sense to try and establish homeopathy and other alternative therapies academically or officially, or whether their outsider status is not the very essence of their role and strength.[63]

Shamanism is a very diverse cultural expression and more than a mere healing method, even though healing is its central function. Originally this term denoted the function of the trance priest healers of Siberian peoples[64], whose special characteristic it is to put themselves into a trance by dancing, drumming or psychoactive substances and during such a trance to visit the upper- or underworld of the spirit beings. In this spirit world they find the solution for problems of the tribe, for diseases or they look for the lost soul of a tribe member.[65] This healing of individuals or the community usually takes place within the framework of a tribal ritual.

People cannot simply become shamans; it is not a profession to be taught, but a vocation which is connected with great privations. Such a vocation often takes place through great dreams or other visionary experiences, which lead those affected far into the realm of illness and madness, into the spirit world, with whose spirits they become acquainted and later acquire their support.

This kind of initiation is regarded as characteristic of shamanism in its original meaning, and there are basic structures of such initiation experiences, visions or dreams that emerge in all cultures. The initiation takes place in an upper- or underworld and is carried out by spirit beings who – in the archetypal form of this process – dismember the shaman and reassemble her or him again. "The novice encounters some divine figures (Lady of the Water, Lord of the Underworld, Lady of the Animals) before he is taken by the animals who lead him to the centre of the world on the top of the Cosmic Mountains, where the World Tree and the Lord of the World is; semi demonic beings discover the nature and treatment of all diseases to him; finally other demonic beings cut his body into pieces, cook them and exchange them for better organs."[66] Thereby he is given new powers with the help of which he can later establish contact with the spirit beings, bring back the soul of the sick or drive away unwanted spirits.

Shamans do not acquire skills merely on the basis of knowledge. Rather, there are personal experiences involved and encounters with spirit beings. On the initiation journey shamans often learn 'their' song, with the help of which they can call the spiritual helpers again or put themselves into an ecstatic state. The drum especially is used for the induction of ecstasy and is therefore sometimes called the 'horse' of the shaman. Animal or plant spirits as well as ancestors are possible spirit helpers. They can also be purely spiritual entities, deities or demonic beings. The animal helpers of a shaman fall under a taboo, that is, they may not be eaten or hunted by this shaman.

The division into upper (heaven), middle (earth) and underworld is typical for the structure of many shamanic world views as well as the world tree in the middle, on which the shaman can ascend and descend and thus move between the worlds. Because of this possibility to move freely between the worlds, the shamans not only have the task of healing and searching for lost souls, but they also accompany the souls of the deceased into the world beyond.

In Hermes (after which hermeticism is named) we see the former shaman god of the Greeks. Hermes was the companion of the dead and wore winged shoes with which he could move in all worlds. His staff with the two snakes looks like a doubled Aesculapian staff (symbol of medicine in Europe) on the one hand, and is interpreted as a world tree symbol on the other hand, the central image for the shamanic world. Hermes was also the trickster, the rogue of the gods; likewise the figure of the shaman is often compared with that of the holy fool.

The concept of 'shamanism' experienced a substantial expansion of its meaning in the course of the last three decades, first from the Siberian peoples to the medicine people and healers of all native peoples, and later also to the modern urban efforts for an expanded healing method reaching into the psychological and spiritual realm and becoming a vehicle of nature-related self-experiences.[67] Thus the term broke away from the connection with indigenous cultures and from the way of healing involving the whole community, which is no longer possible under modern urban circumstances. Only in this more modern sense of the word can we speak of 'shamanism' in connection with homeopathy. By this we mean a form of healing that works through a direct and conscious contact to a spiritual sphere and tries to restore the physical-psychological wholeness of the patients. Furthermore, in this very

98

extended sense 'shamans' are those healers who have a close relationship to nature and its beings and who know how to heal and work on the basis of their own experiences – 'from the guts' as you may say.

One difficulty of modern urban shamanism is that there is no tradition in Western culture of acquiring the personal qualities and learning the skills that make shamans special. Most of those who call themselves shamans today are either autodidacts or have learned from other cultures (mostly the North American Indians). Most of the time their work seems so strange and exotic to average European citizens (if they hear about it at all) that modern shamans can only work within a very small milieu. A typical feature of what we today call 'neo-shamanism' is the use of the drum, with the help of which a more or less deep trance state can be achieved in order to come into contact with the helpers and guides of the spiritual world. Often the people seeking help are taught to find their own 'power animal' or 'guardian spirit' (the shamanic counterpart to the guardian angel) and to establish communication with them. In modern shamanic healing the direct handling of the life energy and the aura also plays a role. And the encounter with trees or other nature beings is sought as a source of energetic healing.

Compared to orthodox medicine, shamanic healing has a creative and unpredictable aspect. The personal element is more important in the healing process and the procedure is less oriented to a system than to the current requirements. This presupposes special qualities in the shamans themselves: they have to learn to give up the idea of a clear cut reality and to move between different levels of existence. What this means for people of other cultures is, of course, difficult for us to understand. But we find again and again reports from members of our culture who have been initiated into a shamanic tradition due to special circumstances. This is reported very vividly in the first books by Carlos Castaneda.[68] Castaneda must learn to transcend his narrow perception and his learned reality in order to spin the threads of reality anew. He learns the connection of all beings: from individuals to community, between community and surrounding nature, between humans and cosmos, between the visible and the invisible sides of the world (consciousness and unconscious we would say in somewhat reductionist terms), between living and dead, between people, animals and spirits, between past, present and future. That makes him another person with special new and often surprising possibilities.

In homeopathic education this shamanic process is not as drastic and profound. Nevertheless, many who have been trained within a mechanistic perspective, experience that they can only gain real access to homeopathy and work with it meaningfully if they allow for very fundamental, new assumptions about reality. Homeopathic education is much more than just learning facts.

A surprisingly large proportion of contemporary homeopaths say that their own serious illness or that of close relatives or some other kind of personal crisis have been decisive in their turning to this path of healing. If we take the very different cultural contexts into account, we can say that today's homeopathic 'medicine men and women' as well as shamans find their vocation through personal initiation experiences. Through experiences that can feel as if one is torn into pieces and reassembled; as if one is immersed in a kind of underworld and returns from it with a new maturity.

Spirits and Remedies

It was not this general context though that led me to look for parallels to shamanism, but the way of dealing with homeopathic remedies.

An essential basic idea of homeopathy is to individualise both the illness and the remedy, i.e. to always start from the individual human being. In everyday practice, however, most homeopathic colleagues do not use hundreds or thousands of remedies, but work predominantly with a certain group of frequently used remedies, the polychrests.

The so-called 'polychrests', i.e. multi-healers, are remedies that are used for very different conditions and frequently. These include remedies such as *Sulphur, Nux vomica, Sepia, Phosphorus, Lycopodium, Calcarea carbonica*. From each of these remedies we find several thousand symptoms in the materia medica. From experience it can be said that about two thirds of the treatments of a normal practice are carried out with about sixty to eighty of these polychrests. For the remaining cases, other, rarer remedies are sought.

It is difficult to explain this phenomenon on the basis of the usual homeopathic theory. First of all, the simple explanation is obvious that this way of prescribing is based on laziness on the side of the practitioners, who do not take the trouble to look beyond their familiar means and really individualise the treatments, as homeopathic theory requires. In some cases, this explanation may be sufficient. For about twenty years, however, there have been intensive efforts to take the demand for individualisation seriously, to expand the limited prescribing practice and to include the many hundreds of potential 'smaller' remedies ['smaller' meaning used less frequently]. And many homeopathy groups all over the world have intensively proved new remedies, which then became their new 'polychrests' for the groups concerned. In spite of all efforts to expand the medicinal treasure effectively, there still seems to be a certain rule that in everyday practice a group of a few dozen remedies emerges which are most frequently used. These remedies can be very different in different homeopaths, which contradicts the notion that certain polychrests in themselves have properties that objectively make them more suitable than others, so-called 'small' remedies, for healing a large proportion of sick people.

It is also a well-known phenomenon that a patient visiting five homeopaths is likely to be prescribed five different remedies, although all five homeopaths have similar training and read the same lists of symptoms and books during the consultation. And this without four of these five prescriptions having to be regarded as erroneous. In a context that relies on science, causality and reproducibility, these examples have to be considered as very suspicious and pointing to a 'dubious' method or to the already suspected placebo effect. How else could it be that the same patient for the same stomach pains gets different remedies from different therapists, all of which are supposed to be more or less effective?

Apart from the fact that in all more complicated cases you would hear five different diagnoses from five orthodox doctors, without anyone questioning the whole of science, the matter is probably different in the case of homeopathy and appears in a clearer light if we take up the comparison with shamanism: shamans get to know a number of spirit beings, which are more or less close and familiar to them, during their initiation and in the following apprenticeship. These spirit beings are the essential helpers in healing and performing magical rituals. Thus a shaman often has a personal protective spirit and more or less many helping spirits, which are known and helpful to him. According to this the power of the shaman is measured.

> "Between the shaman and his 'spirits' a 'familiarity' relationship sets in. By the way, in ethnological literature they are called *spiritus familiaris*, helping spirits or guardian spirits. But it is good to distinguish between the actual *spiritus familiaris* and another, stronger category of spirits, which are called patrons or guides, and these again are to be separated from divine and semi-divine beings, which the shamans call during their sessions. A shaman is a person who has concrete direct relationships with the world of gods and spirits."[69]
>
> "As we have seen, an Eskimo shaman, after his enlightenment, must get his helping spirits all by himself. In general, these are animals in human form; they come of their own free will when the apprentice is worthy. Fox, owl, bear, dog, shark and all kinds of mountain spirits are powerful and effective helpers. With the Alaska Eskimos the shaman is stronger the more spirit helpers he has. (...) From this we can conclude that the guardian spirits and mythical auxiliary animals are not a characteristic and exclusive characteristic of shamanism. These guarding and helping spirits can be won almost everywhere in the cosmos and are accessible to every individual if he only wants to undergo certain quests."[70]

Although homeopaths are not 'initiated', the first learning and assistance periods and teachers are nevertheless formative for a long time. During this time of homeopathic teaching and training, inner images of certain remedies, disease states and treatment strategies are created. These are later refined and corrected, resulting in a group of homeopathic 'spirits' (remedies) to which a practitioner develops an affinity and with which he or she can work most effectively. Often these remedies include those that have been 'proved" and experienced by themselves, as Hahnemann emphasises in his considerations on the homeopathic self-experiment (see box below). In addition, there is then a greater number of homeopathic 'spirit helpers', the so-called 'small remedies', which are used less often and in special cases.

Phatak says in his well-known homeopathic Materia medica: "Drugs should become your friends. You can identify your friend from the way he rings the bell, taps or opens the door, climbs the foot-steps etc. Similarly you should be able to know the drug even when it is partially seen."[71] A homeopathic practitioner becomes really proficient when this level of understanding, this direct intuition for a remedy is reached, when one goes beyond thinking in stereotypes, rubrics (of symptoms) and key symptoms. Only few therapists succeed in this with many remedies – and the spectrum of the therapeutic possibilities depends, like with the shamans, on the extent of this kind of knowledge, to already recognise the remedy by the "tap on the door".

This understanding of homeopathic remedies as spiritual beings that can work in the environment of a therapist who knows them and is 'friends' with them also corresponds to the often made experience that a homeopathic healing process begins already from the moment in which the therapist has come to the appropriate idea of a remedy, the moment, in which 'the case was understood', that is, the personal story of this person's suffering has found connection to a larger understanding and life context.

In summary, it can be said that both shamans and homeopaths work best with the spirits/remedies that they personally know well, that they have seen work in their personal education, that they have experienced in themselves, and whose essence they can often recognise by small things, moods or symptoms that nobody else would notice.

There is a saying that a shaman can only heal those diseases he has gone through himself, or work with those spirits he has known about himself. Hahnemann comes very close to this understanding of the connection between self-awareness and healing when he explains in his main work:

"No true physician can henceforth exclude himself from such attempts, especially on himself, in order to obtain this knowledge of the remedies most necessary to the healing profession, ..." (Organon, §119) "However, those provings of the pure effects of simple remedies in changing the human condition, and the artificial disease states and symptoms which they can produce in a healthy person, which the healthy, unprejudiced, conscientious, sensitive physician himself employs with all the caution and gentleness he learns here, remain the most excellent. He most certainly knows what he has perceived about himself. – Footnote: These self-experiments also have other irreplaceable advantages for him. First of all, the great truth that the medicinal nature of all medicines, on which their healing power is based, lies in those changes of state suffered from the self-proved medicines and in the conditions of illness experienced on themselves by means of the same, becomes an undeniable fact to him. Furthermore by such strange observations on himself, partly for the understanding of his own feelings, his way of thinking and mind (the essence of all true wisdom: gnothi seauton [recognise yourself]), he is formed as an observer which no doctor may lack. All our observations on others do not by far have the attraction than those employed on ourselves. The observer of others must always fear that they who prove the remedy did not feel so clearly what they said, or who did not indicate and name these feelings with the exactly fitting expressions. He always remains in doubt as to whether he is not at least partially deceived. This obstacle to the knowledge of the truth, which can never be completely cleared away when investigating the artificial symptoms of illness caused by medicines in other people, is completely eliminated in self-experiments. The self-explorer knows it himself, he certainly knows what he has felt, and each such self-experiment is for him a new impulse to explore the powers of more remedies. And so he practices himself more and more in the art of observation, which is so important for the doctor, when he continues to observe himself as that which is more certain and not deceiving him, and all the more eagerly will he do so, because these self-experiments promise him the knowledge of the tools which are mostly still lacking for healing according to their true virtues and their true meaning, and which do not deceive him. He also does not believe that such small illnesses would be detrimental to his health at all if he took remedies that were to be proved. Experience teaches, on the contrary, that the organism of the prover, through the increased attacks on the healthy state of health becomes all the more trained in repulsion all enemies of his body from the outside world, and all artificial and natural, pathological harmfulness, and also hardened against all detriments by means of so moderate self-experiments with medicines. His health becomes more steadfast; he becomes more robust, as all experience teaches." (Organon, §141)

As a parallel to this, a statement from Eliade's standard work on the shamanic vocation: "There is nothing surprising about the fact that these diseases almost always appear in a relationship with the vocation to the medicine man. Like the sick man, the religious man is also thrown onto a level of life which reveals to him the fundamental realities of human existence, its loneliness, its insecurity and the hostility of the world around it. But the primitive sorcerer, the medicine man, and the shaman is not simply a sick man; he is above all a sick man who has healed himself. (...) that the selection of the shaman is manifested by a rather severe illness, which generally coincides with sexual maturity. But at last the future shaman recovers with the help of those spirits, which later on will be his protective and helping spirits." (Eliade, pp.37-38)

"What's Wrong with Us?" Healing by Empathy.

This typical medical question is not as ridiculous as it sounds when it is put in the right context: On the one hand, a suffering or a disorder always points to something that is still missing from the whole, from healing. The fact that I, as a sick person, am *missing* something hits the matter much better in depth than the idea that I *have got* something, such as a 'pathogen' or a 'disease'.

On the other hand, *we are* always missing something when a member of the community on this planet is missing something. The modern individualism that makes me think I can be healthy when you're sick is a big illusion. Healing ceremonies of all peoples and times involve at least the extended family, often the whole tribe. In fact, *we*'re always missing something.

Homeopathy sees this connection just like all traditional peoples. The homeopathic art of healing is based – as its name suggests – on the process in which the patient and the practitioner come into harmony, that they each have a different share in a similar suffering.

It only superficially looks like a contradiction if homeopathy in particular wants to individualise more than any other medicine on the one hand, so it regards every suffering as something belonging to the path of life of this very special individual human being, and if, on the other hand, with its therapeutic attitude it emphasises precisely the communal. It thus reverses the polarity common in orthodox medicine at both ends and reverts to a wisdom that humanity has always carried in this respect. Where the special and individual could easily be observed on closer inspection, orthodox medicine generalises the form of suffering into a 'disease'. On the other hand, it isolates the sick and sorts them out as in need of repair from the community of those who are still functioning. Holistic medicine, on the other hand, leaves the sick person within the community and even pays them special attention as carriers of symptoms that affect us all. And it observes the individual peculiarities of this illness very closely and if possible without rough schemata.

Beyond this basic attitude, in modern homeopathy the close connection between people is also used diagnostically. The principle of transference and countertransference known from psychoanalysis and applied in modern psychological therapies has also found its way into homeopathy and has proved its worth here. Transference is understood in the sense that the patients project (transfer) inner images and feelings onto their therapist and experience them in her or his person. In the countertransference, the therapist experiences in her- or himself psychological traits of the patient that have remained unconscious. Depending on the sensitivity of the patient, these consist of moods, feelings or concrete body symptoms of the patient. Transferences and countertransferences occur in principle in all therapeutic processes, but are not always consciously perceived and are not taken into account in many therapeutic approaches. It is part of every good therapeutic training to become aware of such processes and to be able to separate the patient's psychic contents, feelings or images that one is experiencing from one's own. On the one hand, it is important for the practitioners to distance themselves from the content adopted, i.e. not to

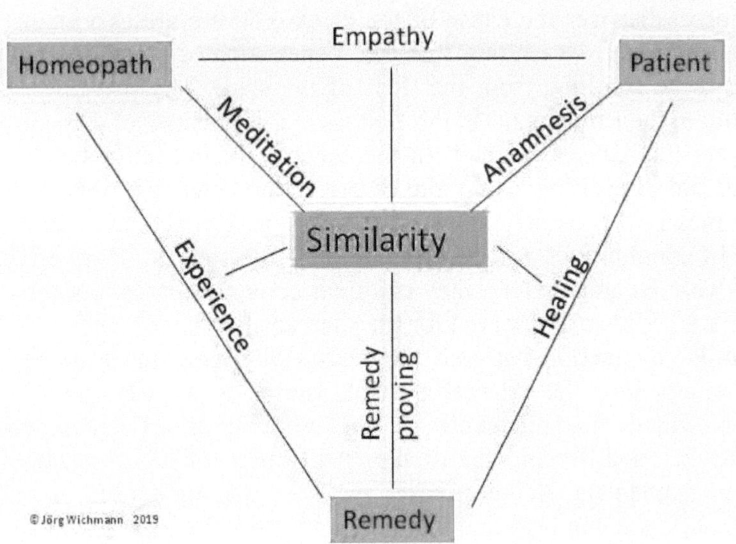

identify themselves with it; on the other hand, the experience of such countertransferences provides extremely valuable diagnostic clues, which often cannot be obtained by any other means. The name of *homeopathia*, of therapeutic suffering and similar suffering, is thus given a special imprint. The shamans' journey into the mental world of the sick is very similar to that of homeopaths – with the restriction that the latter usually do not reach trance states in their work.

The practice of homeopathic remedy provings by the practitioners themselves, the value of which Hahnemann repeatedly emphasised, can also be understood in this context: the practitioners experience the individual and special nature of a remedy on their own bodies and enter into an experiential community with the patients by becoming fellow sufferers (according to the name of *homeo-pathy*).

Shamanic Aspects of Homeopathy

Let's look at a few more parallels between homeopathy and shamanism.

First of all, there is a fundamental concordance in the understanding of disease: "When the shaman is called to a sick person, he first tries to discover the cause of the disease. There are two main types of diseases: those resulting from the penetration of a pathogenic object and those resulting from the 'loss of the soul'. The two differ considerably in their treatment. In the first case, it is a matter of driving out the agent that causes the evil. In the second, to find the patient's flighty soul and insert it back into him or her. In the latter case only the shaman comes into consideration, because only he can see and catch the souls. In communities where, in addition to the shaman, there are medicine-(wo)men and healers, they can treat certain diseases, but the 'loss of the soul' is always reserved for the shamans."[72]

A similar distinction between the causes of illness can also be found in homeopathy: the external ailments caused by a clear '*causa*' and the so-called 'derangements of the vital force'. Of course homeopathy has a different idea of the 'penetration of a pathogenic object' than shamanism. Acute diseases are those that are caused by a trigger, '*causa*', and can heal on their own if they do not lead to death. A chronic disease, on the other hand, does not heal on its own and has a

108

stronger connection to the patient's biography. This chronic derangement of the life force corresponds to the 'loss of soul' in shamanism. Even in homeopathic treatment, the acutely triggered disease states are treated differently than the chronic ones, 'loss of soul'. Depending on how threatening they are, acute conditions are left to the body's ability to heal itself, surgically treated, alleviated with household remedies or treated with a homeopathic acute remedy. The entire individualising homeopathic art of healing is dedicated to the chronic disharmony of the vital force.

> **Jeremy Sherr on Shamanism and Homeopathy**
>
> Jeremy Sherr is one of the few modern homeopaths who is very aware of the inner connection between homeopathy and shamanism. In an interview[73] he says about this connection between homeopathy and shamanism: "Shamanism is a healing art. It's a collective name for the healing arts. But it's based on experience, the personal experience of delving into nature and the darker side of ourselves in order to unite ourselves with nature, our light side with our dark side, our conscious with our subconscious, and to heal the great rift between the male and the female.
> And shamanism employs any trickery possible to do this. Any voyage possible, because it's a personal voyage. It's like the voyage of the hero, of the explorer, of deeper territories, of mysticism and nature. Of the world of potency and imagination, drugs and experience, healing and the subconscious. Homeopathy is a modern shamanism.
> Question: You have said that provings are shamanism.
> Provings are very much the shamanistic side of homeopathy, although there are other sides too, such as the meditation of taking a case. But in provings you are delving into nature, you are taking a trip to the other side. The other side of nature, but the other side of yourself too, a side of yourself that you'll never reach through daily experience. And what's more, you're doing it as a conscious group that's grown together, which makes it much more powerful. You take a collective trip to an aspect of the self and of the universe that has maybe never been touched before in the whole history of humankind."

Furthermore, in the comparison between shamanism and homeopathy, the observance of certain taboos in shamanic healing (food and touch taboos) can be related to the strict avoidance of certain 'antidotes' (coffee, mint, essential oils) in homeopathic treatment. The naming of this particular antidote, which is supposed to disturb the effect of homeopathic remedies, is in many respects illogical and inconsistent[74], but is strongly reminiscent of the accentuation of a healing process by occupation with taboos. Consequently, we also find a less strict adherence to the antidote 'taboos' among those homeopaths who orient themselves less to the 'ritual' of homeopathic prescription, but rather pursue a psychological or spiritual approach, i.e. attach more importance to the awareness of the respective process.

In addition to these similarities, which lie more in the concepts, there are other parallels in practice. When we look at the effect of a remedy, we usually assume that it has to be taken by a person and then begins to work in their body. Such an idea, however, does not adequately describe the nature of a homeopathic remedy. Even in the way it is manufactured and in the way it is prescribed, homeopathic remedies cannot be compared with chemically active medicines. Experiences in homeopathic remedy provings and in practice show that the encounter with the essence of a remedy is by no means limited to the process of material ingestion (and even this is no longer a material one). Hahnemann sometimes only allowed patients to smell the remedy in order to establish contact with it and achieve an effect. Many homeopathic remedy provings today are carried out as so-called 'pillow provings', in which the proving persons place a sachet of corresponding globules under the pillow for one or more nights.

Another aspect of exceeding the material effect and the conception of the same in the prescription of remedies may be illustrated by a small incident from practice, which was reported to me by a colleague: A mother called her from a holiday in Spain, many miles away from the nearest pharmacy and several days of waiting for the next homeopathic remedy. Her two-year-old child had severe diarrhoea with great loss of fluid and became visibly weaker. The therapist came to the conclusion that the child should receive a certain homeopathic remedy (*Podophyllum*). However, this remedy was not at the place of the event and could not be procured. The therapist prescribed one of the remedies

110

that the mother had taken with her, but without effect. Two hours later she prescribed a second remedy, which is often used for bowel problems (*Nux vomica*), but was only moderately suited to the child's condition. However, it was the only one of the remedies at hand that still came into question, but it had no effect either. Since the child became weaker and homeopathically it was clear that it needed *Podophyllum*, the therapist used a 'trick' which she knew some colleagues had used in such emergencies: she had the mother write '*Podophyllum* C30' on a piece of paper, put a glass of water on it and wait ten minutes. The child got sips of the water until the condition improved. The improvement came quickly, and after one day the child was almost healthy.[75]

Such a story would serve critics to disqualify homeopathy or the practitioner, but it clarifies the connections mentioned. Firstly, we see that the effect could not have been based on suggestion, for then it should have had an effect after the first two remedies given with full conviction, not after the last, which was applied with great scepticism and little hope left. And secondly, the encounter with the medicinal essence Podophyllum is obviously not bound to the globules, but can be produced in a purely spiritual way. The material form of the administered medicament, even if it is in the merely symbolic materiality of high potency globules, can thus be completely exceeded in practice.

In the experience of those who take a remedy or carry out a remedy proving, such transgression of the everyday boundaries of individuality and perception takes place as well. Some homeopaths with rich proving experience question the concept of 'remedy proving' because it is too reminiscent of the clinical chemical drug proving of conventional medicine: "We deliberately call it a remedy encounter and not a proving because we encounter the nature of the remedy and this not only makes symptoms (illnesses) visible in us, but also introduces us to ways of seeing and behaving, experiences, events and 'coincidences' which we have not encountered before, or only very rudimentarily."[76] A typical experience with homeopathic remedy provings conducted in seminar groups is that not only those taking the remedy encounter it, i.e. have corresponding dreams or experience symptoms, but also other seminar participants. Even partners at home can experience remedy effects.

The image of a field-like effect is imposed upon us, of a field, which produces a resonance in various places. These 'resonance phenomena' seem to know neither boundaries between individuals nor between the inner and outer worlds, as remedy effects obviously do not only take place on the body, in the feelings or dreams of the provers, but also in the outside world. In the proving of the remedy *Neon*,[77] one of the provers who did not know the proving substance reported that on the day the remedy was taken she found a load of broken neon tubes in front of her house, which someone had thrown there overnight to get rid of.

C.G. Jung coined the term *synchronicity* for such experiences, indicating a meaningful simultaneity of events that are not causally connected. He was often able to observe such 'synchronicities' in therapeutic or other intensively charged situations. For scientifically thinking people, such a thing is merely a 'coincidence' and does not belong in the system of explainable or explanation-needy reality; within a holistic view of the world, such events and contexts are a natural component of perception and expectation of the world. They belong to the basic principles of existence, the occurrence of which we can assume in the same way, as it is natural for scientists that a stone will always fall down.[78]

Another plastic example for synchronous or analogous events is a remedy proving in a larger group during a one-week homeopathy seminar: *Chininum sulphuricum*, a previously little known remedy substance, was proved. Several conspicuous dreams arose among the provers, dealing with accidents in the food sector. One participant, for example, dreamed of a kitchen fire at MacDonalds. Three participants who had not taken the remedy had a strange incident in their apartment: a cable in their fridge burnt so that all the food in it was contaminated and had to be thrown away. This incident got its meaning and context only at the final group meeting through the similar dreams of the others.

Since its very beginnings, homeopathy has also known the direct transfer of life energy. In Hahnemann's day, there was talk of mesmerism or magnetisation. He wrote in 1842: "If one has learned to proceed correctly with zoo-magnetisation/mesmerisation in order to emphasise the intended effects on the sick person, the combination of both, that of homeopathic treatment with duly dynamised well-chosen remedy in appropriate administration, with functional zoomagnetic treatment of the sick person together will only form the most perfect possible way of recovering sick people, which, however, we can only expect after many years have passed".[79] Since Hahnemann was completely aware of the placebo effect and also used it consciously,[80] we can be sure that he did not understand mesmerism, i.e. the transmission of life force by laying on hands or stroking hands, in a suggestive sense, but as a direct, non-material influence of the human organism by a therapist. The use of mesmerism was largely lost within homeopathy when it was sought to be aligned with mechanistic principles. In different forms of spiritual healing, laying on of hands, Reiki and similar therapies the old mesmeric healing magnetism lives on.

Hahnemann explicitly placed himself in the tradition of spiritual healing when he wrote in the *"Homeopathic Memories"*: "Real homeopathic healing is a true cult, a sacred act in which the good homeopath represents the place of the creating Deity in order to transform the human creature corrupted by illness ..."[81] This 'transforming' is a thoroughly shamanic concept, which does not exist in any conventional medicine in Europe. Since we can be sure that at Hahnemann's time there was no conceptual knowledge of what we today call shamanic, it is all the more amazing how exactly he could sense and name the essence of the tradition in which he (unknowingly) put his medicine.

We live in a modern world in which we expect to meet something like 'shamanism' and 'magic' in exotic outer forms. An academic sitting in front of a computer and sending an ordinary bill after the treatment does not fit into our scheme of the shamanic. Yet as soon as we detach ourselves from the outer form and try to discover concordant patterns behind the temporal habits, then we find a great closeness between these healing modes.

Therefore I would like to summarise again, which similarities between the shamanic and the homeopathic way of healing are noticeable and where the differences lie.

<u>self-experience</u>
- that their healing action is based on experience and observation, both in training and in the practice of healing.
- that the healers always make their own experiences with the remedies
- that they experience symptoms on their own body or on their own mind

<u>relationship to the sick</u>
- that they 'travel' with the patients into their inner world / for homeopaths this means to become similar
- that they do not relate to the sick as outside experts but as compassionate companions
- that they use their intuition and sensing in addition to concrete knowledge about connections in the body and about remedies
- homeopathy and shamanism individualise the disease while the patient remains in the community; whereas allopathy isolates the patient and generalises the disease.

<u>relationship to remedies</u>
- the personal way to choose remedies that work better, the better we know them / which is similar to the fact that the shamans must know their spirits
- that they have an intimate and partly personal relationship to their remedies and regard them less as things than as beings
- that their notion of disease and cure is a non-material one.

<u>world view</u>
- that they have a holistic picture of humans and nature and do not divide between body and soul
- a spirit loses its power if one knows its name and performs the appropriate ritual / a disease is cured by naming the remedy and applying its immaterial information (i.e., by a potency higher than Avogadro's number)
- that for them healing finds its meaning only in a larger spiritual context of life

The differences are,

- that shamans usually heal out of a changed state of consciousness and homeopaths usually do not,
- that the self-(mis)understanding of modern homeopaths is predominantly scientific,
- that homeopathy appears to be a drug based therapy (apart from Hahnemann's enthusiasm for the laying on of hands).

Due to the knowledge about the nature of homeopathic healing as presented here, I have been forced in the course of time to abandon the idea of a theoretically clear, rationally teachable and ultimately formalisable homeopathic method, as laid out by many well-known representatives. The image of the homeopath as a magician or shaman who sends out her or his spirits for the benefit of the sick and who does not only have to memorise a pile of books, but also has to instigate profound changes in his or her psychic structure, looks completely different. I assume that a large part of my colleagues will not recognise themselves in this picture – the external form that homeopathic work has taken in the last two centuries is too dissimilar. They have always tried to orient themselves towards scientific accuracy, to achieve a conscientious objectivity of their actions and to satisfy the maxim of the greatest possible rationality. The self-image of all well-trained practitioners is deeply influenced by this tradition. But when I look over my own shoulder and that of other homeopaths and see how decisions are ultimately made about the choice of remedies, about potency, the duration of waiting and so on, the claimed rationality proves to be an apparent one. There is no really logical way to distinguish the important from the unimportant symptoms in the anamnesis, to ask the patient the right questions, not even to find the right remedies in the repertory from the finished case analysis. Jokingly we sometimes say: A well-chosen repertory rubric is one that contains the right remedy! But that sentence really hits the point.

The homeopaths of the past, who had to exist in the environment of a narrow mechanistic world view, and most of today's practitioners, due to their scientific socialisation, need this illusory rationality in order to justify their actions to themselves and others. But they need the

115

'shamanic', their intuition and confidence in the magic of the remedies to be able to heal effectively. Thus homeopathy appears as a form of personal magic, which as such can only be taught to a limited extent. Each and every one must find a way for him- or herself and find 'their own spirits'. The systematic experiences of others and the influence of good teachers are indispensable guidelines and give the work a solid foundation. But Hahnemann's later renaming his central work from "*Organon of the Rational Art of Healing*" to "*Organon of the Healing Art*" probably had its good reason.

With all these seemingly magical aspects of homeopathy, which places it in the framework of a completely different world view together with alchemy, shamanism and esotericism, there is one essential difference that remains: shamans deliberately and controlledly leave the realm of the ordinary world with their own consciousness in order to be able to heal, while homeopaths (in the tradition of the alchemists) only transport their remedies out of the realm of matter by potentisation.

It may seem desirable to expand the consciousness of homeopathic therapists in the shamanic direction in order to give more accuracy to their work. It is true today that hardly anyone can directly perceive the effect of a remedy on the life force. Rather, it must be derived from the feelings and descriptions of the patient. Hahnemann has repeatedly and clearly spoken out against all 'supernatural speculations' and for the exclusive use of prejudice-free perception. But it is precisely this attitude that speaks in favour of extending the unprejudiced *perceptive faculty* of the practitioners as far as possible. At Hahnemann's time it was not conceivable – or at least not arguable – that human perception could also extend to the life force itself. Today, we know from a variety of experiences and from testimonies of other cultures that such perceptions are quite possible. Within a culture in which there are no useful terms for the experiences of shamanic journeys and 'extrasensory' perceptions and no traditional structure for their processing and evaluation, there is a long way to go, which will be lined with misunderstandings and errors. But I am convinced that we will walk this way and make it accessible for others.

"Real homeopathic healing is a true cult, a sacred act in which the good homeopath represents the place of the creating Deity in order to transform the human creature corrupted by illness,.... "

(Samuel Hahnemann)[82]

Homeopathy and the Spiritual Path

With these considerations we come to the last topic of this chapter: Homeopathy is a way to return into the wholeness of life, a way that therapists and those in therapy walk together and can only walk together. Thus homeopathy – like all other holistic healing methods – places itself in a context which we would today call a spiritual one.

The insight that all life is one, that everything is part of a single energy field, of one spirit, is an important prerequisite for understanding homeopathy (as well as shamanism and alchemy), but is also the inherent message of homeopathic activity. Individuality, the individual illness, the suffering alone, are only temporary illusions. The name homeopathy already indicates this: healing occurs when most similar things meet, in the patient, in the practitioner, in the illness, in the medicine, when resonant vibrations combine to form an overall sound. Thus the reintegration of individual suffering into the overall context, into the wholeness of life, takes place, symbolically as well as actually. Disease, the sick, those treating it and the remedies together in rediscovered similarity re-enter the unity from which they had fallen. Healing and salvation meet.

Homeopathy as a medical method refers to another way of looking at life. "Hahnemann actually formulated the law of similarity for homeopathy, but there are many areas in life where it is just as effective. The most important area for us is the encounter with the patient. In order to be able to perceive this similarity also in the finer shading, it is necessary to develop a sense which we would like to call the similarity sense," say two experienced homeopaths[83]. What is to be effective in the individual homeopathic treatment must be experienced and enlivened in the larger context of life, otherwise the method remains dead and empty. It is not a matter of elevating a healing

117

method to a world view. Homeopathy, however, can only be effective and working in its full potential within the framework of such a philosophy.

Psychotherapies, especially deep-psychological and systemic ones, are closest to this approach. They also strive to bring people back into a larger context of life, depending on the school, into that of the greater unconscious or that of the social community. What they have in common is that the individual is healed by expanding her/his too narrow boundary to a greater one. In the case of sick children, it is the family that has to rearrange itself in order for a deeper healing to be possible. First, the energetic disharmony must return to where it came from, usually to the parents. Through this perspective many feel threatened, confronted with their feelings of guilt. But the responsibility for the whole has nothing to do with guilt or blame. It can also be beneficial for parents to be a couple with problems again rather than parents with a problematic child. In terms of homeopathy, this may mean that a child does not necessarily receive the remedy that is most similar to his or her individual condition, but one that describes the tension of the whole family. This in turn results in new solutions for all parties involved.

Despite this similarity with the systemic approach of psycho-therapy and depth psychology, homeopathy goes far beyond this by not only including family and social connections, but also creating wholeness with nature. It is a simultaneous relationship between humans and healing beings from the natural realms. As much as psychotherapy may contribute to overcoming social boundaries, its approach as such manifests a fundamental division of our culture that leads to further continuation of our collective problems. The cultural historian Roszak analyses: "Though it is rarely discussed in the professional literature, Freud's despairing vision of life continues to haunt the major schools of mainstream psychiatric thought. It is a sort of negative presence, unmentioned but always there in the background: the image of a cosmos too alien to take into consciousness. The decision modern psychiatry has made to cut itself off from nature at large and minister to the psyche within a purely personal or social frame of reference follows from Freud's courageous but failed effort to

118

find a humanly acceptable connection between the inner and the outer worlds."[84]

Homeopathy goes a decisive step further and is therefore more comprehensive in its healing possibilities. It does not only build on the relationship between people, but includes the wholeness of life. The world of homeopathy is not just a social, urban world, not just a world of libraries and therapy rooms. The manifold beings of nature are with us in their hundreds, and we have to get involved with them in order to find healing, health and ultimately salvation.

Thus homeopathy can offer a way or support to greater health. Working with the laws described here and with the homeopathic remedies can be used to accompany a spiritual path of development. Hahnemann himself hints at this when he speaks about the effects that the long-term performance of ever new provings has, or when he speaks of the 'transforming' of the whole human personality through homeopathy. Apparently he had more in mind than better functioning in everyday life. Homeopathy can be a spiritual path for the therapist, just as the learning of any holistic form of therapy should be. And it can offer this to those patients who expect more from a therapy than the restoration of their physical functions.

In homeopathy, this path consists of relating to and establishing contact with a wide variety of substances on our planet in various ways – through remedy provings, triturations, meditations or even direct contact. This path, again, is very similar to the originally shamanic one.

There are few people who know so much about so many completely different substances, their history, cultural significance, medical, biological or chemical properties as homeopaths who take their work seriously. But it is not this knowledge in itself but the path to acquiring it that can make homeopathy a path of inner change and maturation beyond a healing method. A fascinating path, which leads not only into the depths of our own soul, but also into the spiritual depths of the world around us, which connects us more deeply with ourselves, with each other and with the world.

"Taking into account the historical development of medicine, however, it is difficult to see orthodox medicine, which was developed relatively recently, as the starting point and other forms of medicine as its supplement."   *(Bruno Rösch)*[85]

Self-confidently Different – Homeopathy in Modern Society

Einstein is supposed to have said that one cannot expect a solution to a problem from the same concepts that led to its emergence. We can apply this insight not only to orthodox medicine, but also to the whole world view, of which it is an offshoot. In the crisis of modernity, which is reflected in the ecological, social and spiritual crises of recent decades, a whole world view and the social, economic and political culture based on it are declaring bankruptcy.

These crises are judged very differently by the people of our culture, since many are doing quite well superficially and a widespread prosperity makes them overlook many 'side effects' of our lifestyle. But our health is unbribable and reflects both by the steady rise in chronic diseases and especially mental illnesses and by the public health crisis that the price for our way of life is becoming more and more expensive. At this point most people become clearly aware of the crisis – especially when they themselves become ill. In the absence of a commitment to any spiritual attitude, health in our Western society has risen to the highest value of personal life, as all surveys show. Therefore, on the stage of health policy, fierce ideological and power struggles are being fought. Although large parts of the population want gentle and holistic healing methods, those responsible for policy exclusively favour technical and chemical medicine.

Given the many side effects and dangers posed by modern medicine, it is easy to understand that many people are looking for real alternatives. Homeopathy offers such a basic alternative. Like other holistic healing methods, it is not just a gentle complement to the established treatment methods, but a fully effective alternative healing system in itself. It has its own methods and goals and is on a par with conventional medicine. However, holistic views and methods and orthodox medicine stand on a completely different ideological ground and contradict each other strongly in their approaches.

In a liberal state, we are prepared to expect to have the right, as responsible citizens, to choose our world view, our science, the way we live our lives, and also our own medical treatment, without being patronised by certain ideologies. In fact, however, holistic healing methods have to justify themselves to representatives of orthodox medicine and have to prove the effectiveness of their methods on the basis of mechanistic standards that are completely unsuitable for this purpose. It is tacitly assumed that the established orthodox science is universally valid as an ideology, objective and valid for all citizens as yardstick. Such a consensus may have existed in Central Europe for several decades, but it disappeared during the 1980s and 1990s. Our society has become pluralistic in the sense that a variety of convictions, beliefs and ways of life may coexist. Only in medicine is there an all-dominant ideology supported by the state. In the course of this book, however, it has become clear that the orthodox view of the world is only one of several possible views, that other views of the world with their medical and scientific methods are also coherent and can draw on a great treasure of experience. Why should the old and proven holistic forms of medicine be judged by the rather young and only in a few generations tested orthodox medicine and accept its supremacy?

A Question of Tolerance

Some people are surprised why such a deep gap opens up in conversations between representatives or followers of orthodox medicine and those of alternative medicine – even up to the level of hostility. Would it not be possible to *coexist* excellently and work together for the good of mankind? With this pious wish it is forgotten that orthodox medicine and holistic medicine are not simply two methods that could coexist. Rather, it is a chasm in world view, science, ethics and the human image that could hardly be deeper. In many respects, the aims of what the respective disciplines strive for are even directed against each other. By 'healing' the one understands the disappearance of unpleasant, senseless and even dangerous symptoms, while the other means the incorporation of symptoms into a greater unity of life, their understanding and their dissolution through acceptance. Across such an ideological crevasse, even mere communication is a laborious task. In addition, communication is made more difficult by an objective power imbalance, since orthodox medicine is preferred by the state and by law. – The present book would like to make a contribution to this frequent misunderstanding, but this contribution can only consist of an honest clarification of the positions.

The demand for a better understanding, for tolerance is easy to set up, but on closer inspection represents an incredibly high demand. In the development of a personal world view, we can roughly distinguish three stages that each individual must attain for himself. The first level of understanding is the naive adoption of tradition. All people get to know a certain view of the world through parents and school, which they have to acquire before further development is possible. For many this level is sufficient; they remain in the learned tradition, which provides them with sufficient tools to get along in the world and to classify their experiences. Once the world view has proved its worth and stabilised, its followers will offer considerable resistance to having the basic structure of their reality questioned. This attitude is natural and necessary. All people initially behave in this way; otherwise there could be no consistent culture.

Some people, however, encounter insurmountable contradictions in the traditional world explanation or have experiences that contradict it – such as encounters with other cultures[86] or personal crises. They rebel against the traditional, feel betrayed by tradition and excluded from a whole realm of reality. The newly emerging world view is initially oriented towards the rejection of the old, and some people even develop an urge to refute the others. After all, the new world view is stable and defended just as the old one was. This, too, is a natural and necessary development that we can observe in individuals as well as in entire subcultures and historically in cultures, such as in the Enlightenment epoch's dealings with Christianity.

The third stage of understanding is insight into the justification of all spiritual directions and tolerance for them. If you mean it seriously, tolerance is the most difficult and can only be achieved through severe internal crises. Our loose tolerance is often based only on not taking everything very seriously and not thinking properly. For a truly convinced orthodox physician who is exposed to the basic questions, it cannot be easy to tolerate homeopathy. In his view, homeopathic practitioners *must* cheat their patients because they clearly and demonstrably give ineffective remedies. Sugar globules *cannot* work according to his view of the world; and he must be convinced that his homeopathic colleagues know this too – after all, they have been trained scientifically like him. If he takes seriously his own theory and experience of the world according to which he works daily, there can be no 'alternatives' to these insights. Admitting that homeopathy *could* work is shaking the foundations of one's own work and one's innermost beliefs.[87]

The deep insight that there can be different world views, which not only superficially or in philosophical abstraction, but up to the practice of life, even into the perception, *see* the world differently, arrange it differently – almost live in a different kind of reality –, this insight is not easy to gain and often much more difficult to bear. Those who follow an alternative path should understand this psychological fact in other people. Someone who does something completely different self-confidently and naturally is more difficult to endure than an ideological opponent within the own system. And it's the serious ones who *have to* defend themselves. The superficial and ignorant will not feel questioned because they cannot even understand and recognise the inquiry as such. Their ignorance is easily confused with tolerance.

The relationship between world views is similar to that of different nations: if one nation were oppressed by another for a long time and not allowed to develop its own culture, then there are always those among them who would prefer to be like the more powerful oppressors and who would seek to adapt themselves. And there are the radicals who would want to abolish the oppressors, avenge themselves and become oppressors themselves. The path to peaceful coexistence, however, does not lead via either path, but presupposes genuine equality. A friendly and peaceful partnership is only possible if the oppressed people can develop their own culture and their own values and ways of life in peace and freedom and if they have gained stability. Only then can they approach each other again and discover which strengths and which weaknesses each other has, how they can complement each other and how they can live together. – For today's predominant orthodox sciences and the alternative world views, this will still be some way to go, but the process has already begun on both sides. On the scientific side, relativity theory and even more so quantum theory have caused such severe ideological upheavals that nothing is as it used to be and much is considered possible.

But no matter how the internal relationship between the mechanistic and the holistic view of the world will develop on the philosophical screen, a secular, pluralistic and democratic constitutional state can always be expected to preserve neutrality and treat all world views equally.

Just as in the clash of Christianity, Islam and Atheism it is true that even the very convinced representatives of the respective groups have to endure that beside them other people have a completely different picture of the world and want and are allowed to live according to it. Thus, in other ideological conflicts, too, the state must keep its distance and guarantee the right of all people "to go to heaven in their own way"[88].

Two World Views and Two Medical Paths	
Materialistic-mechanistic world view	Holistic world view
• world as a random product of atoms, energies and physical laws	• world as an ordered wholeness
• chaos = a universe of random causalities	• cosmos = a universe of meaningful relations
• causal structures only	• analogous and causal structures
• life as a result of chemical-physical mechanisms (reductionism)	• life as an independent phenomenon (vitalism)
• knowledge through measurement and calculation	• knowledge through observation and empathy
• analytical only	• analytical + intuitive – synthetic
• only everyday consciousness valid	• different levels of consciousness
• information for mastery	• understanding for wisdom
• agnostic	• spiritual
"Orthodox medicine" (allopathy)	Homeopathy and holistic healing
• I have a disease.	• I am ill.
• the disease as a starting point	• the patient as a starting point
• pathogens cause the disease	• pathogens colonise diseased tissue
• disease as a malformation	• disease as a path
• symptom as danger or annoyance	• symptoms as a useful guide
• objective symptoms are more important	• subjective symptoms more important
• fear as basic sentiment	• confidence as basic sentiment
• medicine fights and intervenes	• medicine regulates
• illness and death as enemies	• illness and death as part of the life cycle
• doctors as experts	• healers as companions
• technology and chemistry repair	• humans and nature heal
• body and mind as separate	• a unity of body, soul, spirit

Tolerance as a characteristic trait can only be developed and developed with difficulty. But tolerance as a principle of the rule of law must be demanded and be the basis of our policy and jurisdiction.

A Question of Ethics

Of course, tolerance for other approaches is particularly strained in questions of ethics when it comes to decisions for concrete actions with regard to society.

Mechanistic or materialistic science is more than a method to attain knowledge. It is also a matter of mentality, or rather it shapes such a mentality and is thus inextricably linked with many other social processes: The repeatability of experiments (demand for reproducibility) corresponds to the repeatability of goods (assembly line instead of individual craftsmanship) and makes these possible and consistently leads to repeatable humans (genetic cloning).

We must abandon the idea that ethics can be thought of or handled separately from science. Rather, there is an inherent ethic in every way of knowledge and science, whether we like it or not. The ethics underlying modern mechanistic science are those of power, feasibility and repeatability. The invention of the cloned, industrially produced baby is not a misdevelopment and not an abuse, but a development that is as much part of the system as the devastating weapon technology and the poisoning of everything organic. The attempt to retroactively limit an already completed cognitive process through a set ethic is pointless and misses the essence of human cognition and action. The ecologically dedicated are also mistaken in believing that we need a more mature ethic in addition to modern science. A more mature humanity would not engage in such a search for knowledge. The factual ethics of today are a necessary part of materialistic science.

The ancient sciences were much more aware of these interrelationships and thus ethically more mature and reflective. It was always clear to the alchemists that ethics, piety and the development of the soul were an inseparable part of their search for knowledge and wisdom; that their soul development was a golden thread running through their laboratory work. Only the spiritually mature reached the high art of the laboratory and produced the results desired in decades of work. The division of knowledge and action, of science and morality, of mind and hand, of heart and tool, is a characteristic of modernity that only became possible that way and led to the well known devastating consequences. For human cognition and action as such, this division is atypical.

With the setting of such a division of knowledge and values, of acting subject and objects, a fundamental epistemological, and at the same time ethical, decision has been made, behind which we cannot go back and which unfolds its dynamics independently of later evaluations and desires.

So it is a basic question that has to be answered long before scientific methodology comes into play, whether I want to regard living beings as machines that cannot actually be 'ill', but only defective; or whether I see them as living and animated organisms, whose living expressions are always to be understood as language. The moment I define an 'objective' science that leaves everything spiritual and subjective outside, I have already answered the question.

The fundamental questions in medicine are not only about different healing systems and the question of whether I would rather become healthy with injections, needles or globules. Rather, it is about very fundamental decisions about what I consider to be healthy or ill, where in the healing process I want to take which risks, how and when I am prepared to encounter death. The question that has now become public, whether we really want artificially made beings or even humans – and if not, whether and how we could still prevent someone making them – has made it abundantly clear what is at stake here and that questions that were asked too late have actually long since been answered. This is no different in the private sphere and no less dramatic and fateful. Here are a few examples:

Every healing path has its risks, which lie less in the method than in the nature of the disease that can bring us to the limits of destruction and death. Orthodox medicine regards death and acute, violent illness as enemies that should be fought by all means. By means of refined diagnostics, early detection methods, routine checks and drugs that are able to prevent acute physical processes quickly and effectively, it has become possible to reduce the risks of dangerous acute diseases, accidents or impending physical changes such as tumours to an extraordinary degree. In the process, symptoms are also eliminated, which we evaluate in a holistic view as attempts of the body to bring

128

about healing itself. Stopping fever is the best example. Apart from this, we are chemically correcting conditions, the cause of which clearly lies in a misguided lifestyle: blood pressure problems, disorders of the fat metabolism and liver, diabetes, cardiovascular diseases, can often be prevented or remedied by a healthy diet and sufficient exercise. Orthodox medicine thus promotes a way of life that weakens and damages the organism and, on top of that, prevents attempts at self-regulation in order to ensure functioning in everyday life and to avoid pain. The price for this is an increase in chronic illnesses which, although not directly life-threatening, lead to a slow onset of disease which can usually no longer be cured by conventional medicine, but can only be alleviated within certain limits.

Vaccinations are another example of dealing with fears and risks. It is common to have our children vaccinated against as many acute diseases as possible, and there is increasing social and legal pressure on those parents who have a different attitude. And there's a billion-dollar business associated with it. It is indisputable that it was not the vaccinations that led to the disappearance of the major epidemics, but hygiene, nutrition and social improvements. It is difficult to determine whether the risk of suffering permanent damage from the diseases vaccinated against is really higher than from the corresponding vaccination. And anyone who works medically with children in the vaccine age can observe that chronic diseases such as neurodermatitis or asthma often occur after vaccinations. In France, the newly introduced hepatitis B vaccine has even been shown in the courts to be associated with subsequent MS in adolescents[89]. In general, the proportion of chronic diseases in vaccinated populations is higher than in unvaccinated populations. In other words, in the case of vaccinations we accept considerable chronic diseases for a doubtful profit in the area of acute diseases, and the vaccinated children have a much weaker immune system. Nevertheless, it creates enormous fears to run around unvaccinated; fears that apparently have no rational basis.

No one can decide for someone else which path is more appropriate, that of a violent, acute but risky crisis with possible solutions on a deeper level, or that of a slowed chronic development with less risk of imminent death. And we are not always prepared to take the risk of a crisis – at least not in the form of diseases.

Interestingly enough, in our society, which has such a panic about the risks of disease, almost all people are ready without hesitation to take on much greater risks, even with a direct risk of death, in order to have a more comfortable motorised traffic. – All these are not inherent necessities, but life decisions, which we make daily and which determine our everyday life.

Within the framework of conventional medical treatment – and this is completely undisputed – tens of thousands of deaths are accepted every year in every western country due to resistant germs and also tens of thousands of deaths due to the side effects of drugs. If even a few people were to die of acupuncture or homeopathy, a complete ban on these methods would certainly be discussed. Fortunately, there hasn't been a single such case. However, the fact that mechanistic medicine itself is responsible for some of the most frequent causes of death in all rich countries has not given rise to a comparable discussion.

We can observe from such examples that collective ethical preliminary decisions profoundly influence our feelings. And it is very difficult to make a decision for a self-determined path in one's own illness and health. Especially when strong pressure, legal disadvantages and anxieties are to be expected. To obtain information about the ideological backgrounds of our ethical decisions can at least be a first step towards genuine self-determination and maturity.

Homeopathy and its Opponents, the 'Sceptics'

Since its foundation, homeopathy has been controversial. The forefather of the method, Samuel Hahnemann, was not a person to make himself popular everywhere. And his undoubtedly numerous qualities did not include tolerance. He not only insulted his opponents, but also his followers and friends when they criticised him or deviated from his ideas. Something like that has long-term consequences. Homeopathy was controversial in medicine for a long time, even when it was – as in the US in the 19th century – the established and most widespread method. The fact that it was homeopathy that introduced scientific thinking into medicine and for the first time implemented the now self-evident idea that a medical hypothesis had to prove itself 'at

130

the bedside' – as empirical procedures were described at the time – was all too quickly forgotten.

Just to remind you: in Hahnemann's time there was nothing like today's conventional medicine. And it was he who introduced a few things that are now part of the basic stock of good medical and scientific practice:
-   remedy provings with accurate documentation of trials,
-   evaluation of clinical observations and inclusion of the patient's view and experience,
-   humane treatment of people in a state of mental crisis.

What is standard for us today was completely new at the end of the 18th century and in part difficult to even imagine, let alone enforce. Hahnemann stands in several respects for the transition of a mediaeval medicine (of which a medicine historian once said that the greatest chance of survival for the poor of that time would have been that they could not afford doctors ...) to modern medicine as we know it today.

Most of the time the disputes were about medical questions, about interpretations of principles and observations of case histories. It was only gradually that a fundamental critique of homeopathy arose, referring to the very high dilutions and attempting to reduce the effect on the placebo effect. – Homeopathy has lived quite well for two hundred years with these attacks and misunderstandings, having had its ups and downs, and has continued to contribute to the healing of patients.

Recently, however, a new international phenomenon has emerged: There are well-organised attempts to discredit homeopathy as such and to destroy it altogether. The whole repertoire of medial slander is employed with expertise and with great financial expense. The campaign is moving from one country to the next and has now (2018-19) arrived in Germany, where until now a relative calm has prevailed due to the traditionally good roots of natural and alternative medicine in the general population. These campaigns are carried by a group of fanatical opponents of all alternative and spiritual lifestyles who call themselves 'sceptics'.

The following remarks deal with the term as such, but mainly with the quotation marks, between which it is set. We know well or can look it up, what a sceptic in the true sense of the word is. Scepticism is a philosophical tradition which follows the principle of doubting established dogmas and doctrines of their own theoretical blueprint. Scepticism is an important part of the enlightenment era and gave us a large part of the freedom of thought that we are now used to. True philosophy will always carry a good deal of scepticism as long as it understands itself as part of the Socratic way of thinking and questioning.

But those critics of homeopathy who are impudent enough to adorn themselves with the proud title of 'sceptics' are but the exact opposite. They are not doubting the established doctrines or their own beloved dogmas, but the beliefs of others that they can't stand. But to doubt the view of the ideological opponent has nothing to do with philosophical art and the claim of scepticism. To consider one's own opinion alone as right and that of one's opponent as indisputably wrong is at best fundamentalism and at worst populism. A sceptical philosopher directs the sword of critical questioning to himself and not at the other. (Example: a Christian sceptic is one who questions Christian beliefs in order to better enlighten them, but not one who questions Islam or Buddhism.)

As far as the well organized groups of detractors of homeopathy calling themselves 'sceptics" are concerned, they are rather fundamentalist ideologists pretending exclusive validity of their version of a naïve positivism and trying to enforce it in the whole of our society. This kind of belief system is also called *scientism* (as opposed to science) and it is no science. It is the task of science to explain or calculate phenomena with the help of their well defined methods and tools. It is not part of their task to state which phenomena can occur in reality and which cannot. In science, the existence of a phenomenon is determined by observation and not by theory.

For the discussions about homeopathy and other alternative healing methods it is essential not to get involved at all with this false claim of the 'sceptics'. Fundamentalists generally have no interest in an open-ended discussion or in a common struggle for the truth, because they always believe they know it beforehand. Fundamentalists are only interested in eliminating all dissidents in one way or another – depending on their historically based possibilities this happens

132

somewhere between ridiculing and the stake. Today we must understand that there are also fundamentalists of the belief in scientism. They have as little to do with real science as the jihadists with real Islam or the crusaders with Christianity. This kind of scientistic belief is based on the results of 19th century materialistic science and the idea, which was widespread in some circles at the time, of being able to finally explain the world with it. 20th century science has long since overcome these positions, even if this notion has not yet arrived in all textbooks (see also the chapter on homeopathy and materialistic sciences).

Such ideological fundamentalists should in principle not be recognised as sceptics or scientists, but these terms should always be used in quotation marks and it should be pointed out that materialistic fundamentalists are at work here, whose alleged goals (consumer-protection) are just as deceptive as their self-designation. They are pseudo or fake sceptics.

For real scientists, the phenomena caused by homeopathic cures would be interesting and worth researching precisely because they initially seem to elude explanation by current theories. Such observations – so-called anomalies – falling out of the grid of what is already known and predictable have always led to advances and paradigms in the history of science.

An interesting question would still be what motivates these 'sceptic' groups? With so many grave and obvious problems in this world, it seems an extraordinary behaviour needing massive reasons to invest such a lot of personal lifetime, energy and money to vehemently combat such a weakly represented and obviously harmless medical method as homeopathy. I must confess that I do not personally know anyone belonging to such a group close enough to have an immediate impression of the mindset or background for such bizarre behaviour. I can therefore only speculate based on few encounters in public talks and the published material.

So far I have hardly read a single contribution by these 'critics' that would even testify to a minimum of expertise. The so-called 'critics' have quite obviously never dealt with homeopathy, as is usual with factual criticism. A literary critic is someone who reads literature and then expresses her- or himself in a differentiated way, but not someone who is generally against literature and has never read anything before. But that's different with the so-called homeopathy critics. We can conclude from this that it is not a matter of a factual dispute and that therefore even factually well-founded arguments on the part of homeopaths have no meaning at all and are not heard. Apparently it is all about their emotional fight against and exposure of something, that they don't understand and would actually like to banish completely from the face of this world. The aim of their campaigns is not to improve homeopathy by criticising certain weaknesses, but to eradicate it. This suggests that fear (Angst) is an essential motivation. Only when something frightens me do I have to expend energy to banish it from the world. With fear in the background we can also understand that some of the arguments brought forward against homeopathy are so absurd that often we can only laugh out loud reading them. Great fear distorts the perception of reality.

We also know from other contexts that fundamentalisms are fear-driven, which means that the respective opponents are perceived as enemies and as a completely oversized threat. Since the imagined threat appears as a reality in the distorted subjective perception, however, the fear as such does not become conscious at all and one's own behaviour appears rational and appropriate to those affected. Rational discussions do not help in such a situation.

Besides the convinced fundamentalists who have to defend their scientistic world view with all their might, there are of course lots of freeloaders who can easily play their way to the forefront by advocating a view that is about to become popular and is hyped in the media. They exist in every popular trend and are not specific to our issue; a real objective discussion is naturally not their thing either.

It is obvious that the public defamation of a healing method that is very popular, very cheap and very effective and does not fit well into the established framework of medical technology and chemistry, is very accommodating to some powerful stakeholders. I do not know whether and in what form these pressure groups take advantage of the fears and fanaticism of some fundamentalists and make these small groups appear more significant than they are through funding or media enhancement. It seems obvious to me, but since I have few possibilities to research this, I can only name a few traces.

Back to the question of what might motivate people to invest a lot of time and energy in making life difficult for others who have done nothing to them. Alternative healers only want to do their job and offer medical help to those who want it. They do not missionise and do not want to convince anyone of their method or their view of the world, at least not without being asked and not aggressively. Why do groups of people organise themselves to discredit alternative medicine? Even fanatics and muddleheads need a motive and – if they invest a lot of time – also a financial basis.

During my search for targeted manipulations in Wikipedia I came across an interesting interview with a young woman who took part in the 2018 GWUP conference as a newcomer. The GWUP (Society for Scientific Investigation of Para-sciences, more or less a branch of the American CSI - Committee for Skeptical Inquiry) is the most important society of so-called sceptics[90] in Germany, i.e.: of fundamentalist materialists, who fight in the name of science against everything, which they cannot or do not want to understand. In addition to homeopathy and all other medical methods outside a very narrowly understood mechanistic medicine (in which even a normal doctor would not feel particularly comfortable), this also includes all other alternative or spiritual world views and life styles.

When I read the title of the interview "Homeopathy, Conspiracies & Glyphosate: The Recipe for SkepKon 2018",[91] I became very alert. What does glyphosate have to do with the ideas of these pseudo-sceptics? A glance at the programme[92] showed that in a two-day conference half a morning was indeed dedicated to the advantages of glyphosate and genetic engineering. Moderators of the conference were Norbert Aust and Natalie Grams, the most prominent German pseudo-sceptics, who usually insist on Evidence Based Medicine. Now little in medicine is as well documented with evidence as is the danger of glyphosate. Even the EU Commission, which is certainly not suspected of making lobby-hostile policies, could not escape the evidence. If now the GWUP grants a broad platform to Monsanto advertisement, although the topic does not fit at all into its framework, that makes you sit up and listen. Of course it is quite far from me to spread conspiracy theories here, haha, but how blind would one have to be, not to think very carefully that a connection is possible here....

One should also know that the CSI, Committee for Sceptical Inquiry, the American parallel to the GWUP did not only organise lectures against alternative medicine, but particularly created an organisation, in order to manipulate the large online encyclopaedia Wikipedia in its sense. This organisation is called GSoW (Guerilla Scepticism on Wikipedia)[93] – no joke; and it specifically trains people to manipulate Wikipedia in a skilful and strategically planned way. [94]

If we look at these connections, then the question of who we are dealing with will definitely be answered. Without having to speculate ourselves, we can read directly from the publications of the 'sceptics' that the manipulations of Wikipedia are not part of a broad public opinion-forming process – as was once the original idea of this largest encyclopaedia of mankind – but that this is done by specially trained groups and networks who learn to abuse the open structures of Wikipedia for their own purposes.

Considering all this it becomes obvious that it is not about evidence and science, but about corporate interests that try to oppose any evidence. It is said in all seriousness that glyphosate is healthier than meat, coffee or beer[95] – perhaps the 'sceptics' should not drink harmless *Arsenicum* C30 for public evidence, but a bottle of evidence-based healthy glyphosate. Cheers!

One last observation: the main topic of the conference was no longer homeopathy, but osteopathy, the ineffectiveness of which was to be proven. My frequently expressed assumption that homeopathy is only the first in a line of those to be defamed seems to be confirmed.

To put it in a nutshell: The self-designation 'sceptics' on the part of the organised opponents of homeopathy is factually wrong, testifies to philosophical ignorance and is presumptuous.

Why? Scepticism has a long philosophical tradition in the West and describes a way of thinking that constantly questions itself. Sceptics in the right sense of the word raise doubt to the most important tool in ideology, namely doubt about one's own position, which is thereby clarified more and more in a kind of hermeneutic circle and can approach the truth. The mere doubting of an opposing position has nothing at all to do with scepticism, but is the exact opposite: ideological thinking at bar-room level. Those who try to bring themselves into conversation here as 'sceptics' are indeed dogmatists of a fundamentalist scientism.[96]

I would like to emphasise that I am very interested in a competent, critical and constructive discussion in homeopathy. One of our greatest weaknesses is the fact that such an internal factual debate hardly ever takes place.[97]

It is also important to bear in mind what a mechanistic view of the world, or – as the groups concerned like to euphemistically term it themselves – a 'naturalistic" view, contains as an image of mankind and life as such. In this world view, humans are machines just like all other living beings. Since spirit and soul are not intended in this concept of reality and every personal experience is reduced to an illusion caused by chemical and electrical processes in the brain, there is nothing left of us as human beings but a complex group of molecules that has randomly arisen in a meaningless universe.

In this gruesome perspective of reality, medicine has but the task of repairing defects in these molecular clusters that we mistake for animated beings. To see more in humans than particularly complex machines is considered irrational by the representatives of this view and is not compatible with their understanding of 'science'. Not only homeopathy would fall by the wayside, not only other alternative medicine, but any humane view of the human being. Terms such as dignity, ethics, character, affection, love lose all meaning in this picture of the world, because they cannot be described mathematically and cannot be measured.

On closer inspection, there is no question of how homeopathy is evaluated, but whether we want to reduce ourselves to machines or whether we want to regard humans as beings with soul and dignity. Humanism itself is at stake here.

The End of the Mechanistic World View

A completely unexpected development, contrary to the attacks on non-material views, is currently taking place in philosophy, especially in scientific theory and – based on this – in ontology (metaphysics).

A group of scientists around the IT expert Bernardo Kastrup[98] openly challenges materialism (physicalism) as a possible basic theory for the interpretation of the world. And this not because of ideological or religious concerns, but because it does not do what a good theory should do: provide a coherent and consistent explanation for all known and scientifically described phenomena.

Kastrup proposes an idealist ontology that makes sense of reality in a more parsimonious and empirically rigorous manner than main-stream physicalism (= materialism), bottom-up panpsychism, and cosmo-psychism. The ontology proposed by him and some of his colleagues also offers more explanatory power than these three alternatives, in that it does not fall prey to the "hard problem of consciousness"[99], the combination problem, or the decombination problem, respectively.

His thesis can be summarised as follows: **There is only cosmic consciousness**. We, like all other living organisms, are but dissociated subpersonalities (*alters*) of cosmic consciousness, surrounded by its thoughts. The inanimate world we see around us is the extrinsic appearance of these thoughts. The living organisms we share the world with are the extrinsic appearances of other dissociated '*alters*".

What is special about Kastrup is that he argues very precisely and logically, point-by-point, and not only appeals to a general prior understanding or metaphysical convictions. He attaches great importance to the fact that his theory explains the empirical findings both from quantum physics and from neurophysiological research well and simply.

He presents this point of view so logically conclusively and clearly that we can assume that materialism (or physicalism) in all its variations, which is currently still regarded as 'scientific' in ideological discussions, has been fundamentally refuted and that its suitability as a scientifically meaningful explanatory principle for a comprehensive understanding of the world is disproven.

138

Even though this point of view has so far only been discussed in small scientific circles, its importance cannot be overestimated. For here the mechanistic system, from which up to now only the fatal effects have been deplored, but which still seems to possess an ideological plausibility, begins to dissolve from the core.

In contrast to other scientists such as Rupert Sheldrake, David Bohm or Fritjof Capra, Kastrup does not argue from a marginal position within the scientific community, but from its centre. Since Kastrup has made it his task to refute materialism by means of its own methods and criteria and to carry this out in a brilliant manner, he thus becomes unassailable on an objective level. He argues exclusively from the internal logic of the system and uses only generally accepted scientific knowledge. All his articles he publishes in renowned, peer-reviewed scientific journals.

Of course, the refutation of one theory is not yet proof of another. But the reference to the necessity of proving every assertion on the basis of a mechanistic understanding of the world has lost its justification once and for all. Ontology, epistemology and theory of science will now have to reorient and reposition themselves, as long as they want to stay on an up to date level of scientific and philosophical development. In this process of forming a new paradigm, those disciplines that did not fit into the old paradigm will have an interesting role to play.

Even if there is not yet much to be seen of this at present, this development will also bring about major changes in society and, first in the academic and scientific environment and then in wider circles, will bring about a considerable rethinking and reorientation.

Health Policy against Human Rights

Apart from philosophical understanding remains, of course, the question of political and social power relations. At present, this lies with the academically established materialistic science and the 'conventional medicine' being part of it. It also has control over ideological competitors. Those who do not conform to its rules do not receive any state licenses or approvals and thus no permission to practice a healing profession, no social recognition and no money.

However, Article 9 of the European Convention on Human Rights states:
"(1) Everyone has the right to freedom of thought, conscience and religion; this right includes freedom to change his religion or belief and freedom, either alone or in community with others and in public or private, to manifest his religion or belief, in worship, teaching, practice and observance." And the German Basic Law formulates in a similar way: "(1) All human beings are equal before the law. (3) No one shall be disadvantaged or favoured on account of his sex, descent, race, language, homeland and provenance, belief, religious or political convictions".

So here we are expressly talking about free religion *and* ideology as well as about their *practice.* Since dealing with the body, suffering and death are part of the direct exercise of a philosophical conviction, the discrimination of holistic philosophies and healing methods by the state in research, teaching, admission to the profession and legal practice constitutes a clear violation of the aforementioned fundamental rights. The possibility of a constitutional complaint must be considered here in order to enforce the freedoms guaranteed by Human Rights and the Basic Law in practice.

An example of such discrimination can be seen in the fact that a therapist is regarded as a 'danger to public health' in the sense of the German Heilpraktikergesetz (law about non-academic medical practitioners) if he or she has insufficient knowledge of conventional medicine, but not an orthodox physician if he or she has insufficient knowledge in holistic medicine. – This makes it clear that the state makes a determination which of the world views represents the 'truth' and which does not. Thus people are given preferential legal treatment or are even disadvantaged on the basis of their ideological convictions, even though the Human Rights Convention and the Basic Law clearly prohibit it.

For the benefit of citizens, it is up to the state to protect them from dangerous treatment methods. However, the question is which criteria are used to determine a hazard. A pluralistic state must not use a single ideology as a yardstick for judging and condemning a competing one. Scientific proofs in the conventional sense are not 'objective' and 'true', but results of a preliminary ideological decision, one among several possible interpretations of the world. Within orthodox science these criteria may have their validity, but not for other healing methods.

Further examples of such unlawful discrimination are: the distribution of research funds; the different or lack of rewarding of different methods of treatment by the statutory health insurances; the unilaterally state-subsidised training of medical doctors in orthodox medicine.

In principle, it is not in accordance with the constitutions of free democratic and ideologically neutral or pluralistic states and the human rights conventions for a government to establish ideological or religious truths as valid or invalid through its legislation or to make the representatives of one philosophical or scientific direction or ideology judges over the others. Nevertheless, this is hitherto unchallenged practice throughout Europe and most countries of the world.

Two things will be necessary to change this state: On the one hand, representatives of the established materialistic sciences and orthodox academic medicine will have to become familiar with the idea that the teaching they represent and consider to be true is not the only truth, but one among different ideologies or world interpretations, and that others in society want to claim equal rights for their views. On the other hand, the representatives of the holistic and alternative world views and healing methods will have to consider evaluation criteria for their disciplines and bear the responsibility for their work before their own committees. Complete self-responsibility and equal cooperation with other sciences presuppose much that has not yet been developed – at best there are the first approaches[100]. The role of a democratic, pluralistic state is to make it possible for different world views to coexist on an equal footing and transparently for the citizens.

There is a need for action in the following areas because fundamental rights are not respected here:

- Those who wish to receive medical care in accordance with a holistic philosophy of life are at a disadvantage under social law, i.e. compared with the statutory health insurance funds.
- In terms of professional law, those whose medical training focuses on a holistic discipline are disadvantaged because they have to prove knowledge in the field of the prevailing competitive science in order to qualify, whereas the opposite is not the case.
- In terms of education policy, all holistic forms of science, medicine and ideology and those citizens who do not follow the prevailing orthodox science, are disadvantaged in their practice. Neither in schools, nor in universities appropriate training contents are offered. Research funds are allocated unilaterally according to ideological criteria, because the definition of being 'scientific' is only awarded to representatives of one form of it.
- Regarding any legal questions and in liability law, in all conflicts as to what is to be regarded as a health hazard, which intervention is sufficient or correct, when a duty of care has been complied with and when not, only an expert opinion according to conventional science or medicine is obtained.

A Medicine for the Future

In order to take the first steps in the direction indicated, a new self-confidence of the alternative physicians is essential. This appropriate self-confidence can follow from a historical and ideological self-image that has been put back on its feet. It is not the holistic medicine that still has to prove its 'scientificness', it is on the contrary the mother, the grandmother and the great-grandmother of the young mechanistic fashion trend, and it is not utterly happy with what has become of its grandchild. And these, the mechanistic sciences, will still have to find their place among the proven traditions of mankind. As is the essence of the holistic attitude, the representatives of the more comprehensive healing methods are open to it, but there is still a long way to go before the one-sided mechanistic disciplines have become an integral (and harmless!) mosaic stone in the overall picture of the human sciences.

But what could medicine look like in the future, if there is a desirable ideological equality of the different healing methods? Will there be different medical sects among which confused laypeople will have to choose? Maybe there'll be some confusion for a while. Ultimately, however, a new equilibrium will settle in, in which different forms of medicine assume different roles in the provision of care to the population. All can then benefit from the wealth and diversity of medical cultures created in human history, and each mode of healing can be used in the way that best unfolds its potential, and be complemented by others where they have their greater strengths.

The various medical schools will each develop their own training, examinations and quality criteria, so that everyone can understand what they want to get involved with or commit to. As the case may be, different directions of holistic medicine will provide the main health care, while orthodox medicine shows its strength in specialised diagnostics, intensive care and surgery.

On the basis of what has been said so far, what kind of model of medical care can we imagine to be meaningful and desirable? – The model should be based on good basic medicine consisting of 'household remedies' and easy-to-handle palliating or relieving procedures that can be applied by the patients themselves. Often the best thing is to do nothing and let the organism heal itself. But that's the hardest part to our mentality today. Taking a sledgehammer to crack a nut seems to us to be the most natural thing today. We approach minor disorders immediately with the entire arsenal of intensive care medicine, as if having to save a human life from athlete's foot or headache.

Where the self-healing powers of the organism are not sufficient or can no longer be stimulated, where organic control systems have perished or are not applied at all, it is necessary to keep the organism alive with technical or chemical aids, if one wants this. Never before has medicine been as successful in this field as modern mechanistic medicine is today. Furthermore, it offers incredible diagnostic possibilities that have greatly expanded our understanding of the biochemical processes in the body. However, for cost reasons and because of the strain on the body often associated with this, it should be considered whether each individual diagnostic measure actually contributes to a better therapy. Although we often gain fascinating insights into the body of the diseased person, we are still unable to help him take any further steps.

The holistic healing methods should play their role in the interplay of deeper problems and more serious illnesses. Homeopathy is the most differentiated form of medicine – conventional or alternative – available to us today, alongside traditional Chinese medicine (as long as it is not reduced to acupuncture). This differentiation and complexity should also be taken into account by giving it a place in our health system.

Weighing up the strengths and weaknesses of different medical disciplines and their areas of application, it is not a matter of applying them side by side and simultaneously. Rather, it is a matter of complementing each other in different problem areas. A sensible order within the medical procedure would be:

- In the case of infections and disorders, there is nothing to do at first, but to give yourself rest, to eat more sensibly, to stop using drugs (especially alcohol and cigarettes) and to give the body a chance to heal itself.
- For mild illnesses that last longer than two to three days, use household remedies such as compresses and wraps, herbal teas, sweating, fasting, bed rest, etc.
- Pregnancy and birth belong in the hands of midwives whose experience and expertise stretches over millennia of human civilisation. Being pregnant and birthing children is a precious part of life and no illness at all and needs neither permanent laboratory control nor intensive care.
- In the case of severe infections with no tendency to self-healing or chronic conditions, further diagnostics must first be undertaken (orthodox medicine with laboratory and technical examination methods has an irreplaceable place here). Then therapists should be called in who have a differentiated and holistic therapy method tailored to the individual case.
- Accidents and life-threatening acute situations are the actual field of orthodox medicine, where it can intervene in a short-term manner by means of surgery, antibiotic or anti-inflammatory measures.
- In the case of the most serious illnesses leading to death, it depends on the individual case whether homeopathic or chemical relief or acupuncture promises more success if a cure can no longer be sought.
- In the final stages of illness and life, where intensive care still takes massive technical and chemical measures that only disturb the transition from physical life, it would often be best to again do nothing.

Overall, such a graduated medical approach would be much more cost-effective. In particular, the first two stages of disorders and minor illnesses do not require the help of specialists. An improved medical education of the population about meaningful prevention and healing of simple illnesses, as well as an education to naturalness and calmness in dealing with one's own body, a combination of more knowledge and more trust would be a clever alternative to highly technical, expensive diagnostics and therapy of everyday ailments. Such a health education could start at school, where even today young people learn more about antiquity, equations or galaxies than about the basic functions of their own bodies.

At present, no one among the decision-makers seems to have any real interest in saving money in the health sector and thus reducing the profits of the pharmaceutical industry, insurance companies, the medical technology industry and the medical profession. Everyone knows how easy it could be to save. All previous studies show that alternative treatments are much cheaper than conventional medicine, that psychotherapies bring considerable long-term savings compared to chemical treatment, that home births are less risky and cheaper than those in hospitals, and so on. Against their better judgement, the political will for real change is lacking here because too many earn too much from the current state of disaster. This situation is likely to change only after a complete bankruptcy of the health care system.

This makes it all the more important to know that there are alternatives that not only promise cosmetic changes to what already exists, but also offer fundamentally different approaches. Alternative medicine is not about an additional luxury; it is not part of the wellness area, which we can only afford when there is abundance. Alternative medicine is a sensible, cost-effective, low-risk and sustainable form of basic medical care.

Homeopathy as Sustainable Medicine

Homeopathy is an ideal form of therapy for a different, sustainable, solidary global culture, as it is:

- sustainable, because it requires only minimal physical resources
- decentralised, because anyone can produce and prove the remedies anywhere
- cheap, because the remedies cost extremely little and only human effort is necessary to use them
- global, because its principles can be understood by all and in every culture
- non-linear and open in its approach, because it involves all facets of the human mind and spirit
- holistic, because it has in view the whole human being and its living conditions
- scientific, because it is based on experience and clear principles
- peaceful, because it does not declare war on diseases, but goes along with the process as applied compassion (homoeo)
- strengthening, because it supports and stimulates the organism's self-healing powers
- independent, because almost no technology, no laboratories and no money are needed for its application
- natural, because it mainly uses substances from nature
- spiritual, because it is based on timeless spiritual laws
- simple, because its principles can be understood by anyone with an open mind
- post-modern, because it is open to a multi-layered and pluralistic world view

These qualities and principles can be seen not only as a healing method for human individuals, but also as a model for a different, healthy and workable approach to the world.

In view of the fact that, in the rich countries of the world, medicine is by far the largest turnover factor in gross national product alongside armaments, it becomes clear how important sustainable medicine is for a sustainable, climate-friendly civilisation.

Homeopathy is a healing method that moves between the worlds of modern science and the traditional holistic paths and can contribute good things from both sides. An accuracy of observation, documentation, and resource knowledge has been developed, as well as an international exchange of experience as known only from the materialistic sciences. And it builds on the depth of the intuition of the practitioners, on the direct encounter with the inner essence of the remedies, with their spirit, and an understanding of the totality of life as only the shamanic traditions cultivate. Only those who see both sides can really understand homeopathy and practise it in the fullness of its possibilities.

The confrontation with a completely different kind of medicine, science, way of thinking and lifestyle, which we do not find on a distant exotic island but in the middle of western thinking and everyday life, could give a decisive impulse to the Western cultural crisis. We have known for a long time that Western science is stuck in a mental impasse and can no longer cope with the upcoming questions and crises. This inability extends from basic research to ethics and politics – a culture reaches its limits. These limits are not only factual, but also spiritual – and the inability to recognise this connection as a necessary one belongs to the core of the problem. Since the ecological, social and economic problems facing our world today are nothing more than the outward expression of our spiritual attitude, a solution within the framework of the current system is not even conceivable. The impetus must – as Einstein's quote at the beginning of the chapter says – come from outside, from a completely different way of approaching the world[101], or from within, from the wisdom about the world and the life that people have always known.

Homeopathy in the Context of the Global Crisis[102]

If homeopathy is to contribute to the healing of patients who have to live under conditions, that make them ill, then homeopaths also have to participate in the healing of the whole system. They can and should bring their diverse experience in crisis management to bear in a wider context. Homeopathy can serve as a model for a sustainable art of healing in many respects.

If holistic medicine sees itself as part of a global movement of people working on change, it will also lead to its being perceived differently.

Homeopaths work daily with crises, with individual crises or those of couples and families, focusing on their health and relationships.
But do they also have anything to say about the comprehensive crisis in which our culture and the global world find themselves? Something to say as homeopathic? And is it part of their role and work to do so? – Yes, of course they have, and they absolutely must have.

There are three basic questions on this subject:
1. Is there a larger context for homeopathy, and how does it affect our way of healing?
2. What does the perception of this crisis mean for the public role of homeopathy?
3. How can homeopaths contribute to the healing of the global crisis and what can our contribution be?

1)   Is there a larger context for homeopathy, and how does it affect our way of healing?

At the historical starting point of homeopathy, the *Organon* of Samuel Hahnemann, the first and most important paragraph states:
§1 – The physician's highest and only mission is to restore the sick to health, which is called healing.

149

In view of this sentence, the first question that arises is what Hahnemann meant by health. Does 'healthy' mean that we can again function better as a cogwheel of the large machine and are again reliable workers in the service of others? Is it our intention to repair our patients for better function and availability? 'High mission' or 'highest call' is a great phrase[103], at the side of which Hahnemann elsewhere (§9) puts the sentence "that our indwelling, reasonable spirit can freely use this living, healthy tool for the higher purpose of our existence". Having such a mission to serve the higher purpose of our existence points to a great task that demands all our strength and full commitment. Restoring the sick to health means that we also take part in restoring this world into a place where health can exist. Restoring the sick to health in an insane world is like trying to light a candle under water.

Like allopaths, homeopaths concentrate entirely on treating the complaints of individual people. They speak of holistic treatment, but the wholeness they look at is only an individual. It is clearly our 'mission', our calling, our profession to do more and to make sure that we ourselves and our patients understand what health really means. Just as peace does not consist solely in interrupting the actual fighting, so health does not consist in the immediate cessation of the presenting complaints – however pleasant and important this may be in individual cases. For as little as we can heal the stomach of an altogether ill person alone, as little can we heal an individual person who is part of a sick society.

To put it more abstractly: Health is a systems concept. There is no health of a single part when the whole is sick – that is a trivial thought, and we tend to think: we know all that, why does he tell us that? I mention it again because we 'know' all this only on a very theoretical level, but we practically do not take it to heart and draw no conclusions from it or act accordingly.
Knowledge that doesn't change anything is useless.

The term homeopathy itself already points to the core of what I am about: to heal something similar with something similar – we are part of and similar to what we heal with. We work with substances of this Earth – salts and crystals, flowers and tree bark, animal milk and

150

feathers – and by doing so, we create stronger bonds to our planet and acknowledge that we are basically identical. We and the Whole, Humans and Earth. The division exists only in the confusion of our mind; and by working homeopathically, we take a first step towards its healing.

To look at this from a different perspective, we can also talk about the modern concept of sustainability, which has become a key concept in many sciences, and for good reason. So we can ask ourselves whether homeopathy is a sustainable healing method? If we look at the extremely economical consumption of resources (less than C 10,000 is hardly possible, haha), then this is certainly the case. But is homeopathy also sustainable in the sense of Hahnemann's "lasting restoration of health" (§2)? How can our cures be permanent as long as we have to send our patients back into conditions that have made them ill in the first place? A sustainable method of healing – or, in Hahnemann's words, one that aims at lasting restoration of health – must also look at and take into account the wider context.

If we really take this further paragraph from the *Organon* as homeopaths, doctors, therapists or healers seriously, then we are apparently not only called to cure symptoms and make sick persons healthy, but to know and eliminate "the things that derange health and cause disease". This is indeed an enormous task; one could say, THE task of our time, and certainly far too great for individuals. That is why we are also called to participate as a community and to join the many who are already working on it. Only then can we rightly call ourselves "preservers of health ".

Hahnemann expressly does not speak here of the sick as in §1, but of "healthy people" to whom homeopaths have to render this service. They should therefore ensure that people can remain in a healthy state before an illness even comes into play.

The polluted air that we breathe, the plastic that we constantly ingest with food, the destruction that we constantly have to see, the suffering of countless living beings that our subconscious permanently perceives, are certainly much greater 'obstacles to healing' than coffee or the wrong toothpaste. In order to be good homeopaths, good healers, we need to see the whole context and take our responsibility in it: making and maintaining the whole system healthy.

2 – What does the perception of this crisis mean for the public role of homeopathy?
Talking about crisis, let us also have a look at the crisis in which homeopathy is to be found (2019). After a big boom of all alternative ways of living and healing in the 80s and 90s we are experiencing a general decline and additionally a special animosity towards homeopathy.

With the rise of more and more criticism (or rather pseudo-criticism) of homeopathy, many of the doctors and alternative practitioners affected initially reacted thus: "We must work better, we must follow our method more closely, we must publish more cured cases, we must all speak with one voice, we must provide more scientific evidence", etc. – The point is only: even if they managed to do so, yes, even if they could do *all* of it, the opponents of homeopathy would not even notice. They wouldn't be interested because they are not interested in a genuine discussion at eye level anyway or in a mutual understanding of the respective arguments.

The factual background shows that in the second half of the last century the materialistic mainstream was doing quite well, technology developed rapidly, the last white spots of the planet were subjected to industrial use and exploitation, oil and minerals still existed in abundance, the economy flourished predominantly, and only the well-informed knew about the catastrophes looming ahead. In such an atmosphere, the materialist establishment could comfortably afford to endure a small bunch of crackpots who spoke of wholeness and alternative life, of Love not War, and who preferred esoteric healing arts such as Chinese medicine, shamanism or homeopathy.

But the clearer it became that the common way of dealing with our planet and with human communities would lead to a global crisis, the more intolerant the system became. Now, after a long liberal phase, we

152

are facing a massive ideological rollback, and homeopathy is suffering the same setbacks as all other alternative areas.

Obviously, it is not a question of homeopathy not being able to prove its quality. Rather, it is that it has been identified as dangerous by the establishment, both philosophically and – much worse – economically. What would happen if the medical and pharmaceutical establishment were to admit that there is a medical alternative that is very effective and very cheap and that is easy to practise anywhere in the world and based on a very different understanding of disease and health? Do you really think that would ever be admitted or even hinted at?

So if all our previous efforts at recognition have not taken us where we wanted to go, then it is not a matter of trying even harder, but of understanding that we have moved in the wrong direction. When we look at our overpowering opponents, the self-proclaimed guardians of scientistic dogma, the pharmaceutical companies and health policy, we should not ask ourselves what we have done wrong to provoke their animosity, but we should see that we must have done something very important *right*. Earning the enmity of those who ruin our health, poison our planet and put profit before solidarity is a good sign that we stand and are perceived as standing for the opposite values. This simply means that our efforts to be recognised by orthodox medicine will lead to the opposite of what we want to achieve. The better we can prove the quality of homeopathy, the more vehemently they will fight us because our view of the world is exactly contrary to that of the prevailing powers.

For homeopathy, it will only be one way to talk to those who have an open interest and to address the general public, which is to a large extent still attached to it. And if it turns out that the mass media are too strongly influenced by materialists, or even in their possession to report in a fair way on holistic medicine, then the way must lead through the social media and through a smarter and more effective way of using them.

In the long run, holistic medicine will prove to be the forerunner of a growing and more comprehensive vision of the world and health. It is not modern science that is against it, but only a dogmatic and scientist misunderstanding of it. Science is fundamentally in favour of us. Clear thinking and the achievements of Enlightenment are the basis of homeopathic work. We can relax and trust that truth will always prevail in the long run.

3 – How can homeopaths contribute to the healing of the global crisis and what can our contribution be?
In the 20th century we lived for a long time with the metaphor that it was five to twelve when it came to the environmental situation. Now, in the 21st century, it's past twelve already. We have gone too far and we know that the consequences of our past decisions will catch up with us no matter what we do or do not do now. At best, we can alleviate or aggravate the consequences. Climate change is already in full swing, oil and other resources are already running short, water will soon prove to be one of the biggest problems, and we will soon face an economic crisis against which the last one of 2008 was only a small foreplay.

How would a 'treatment' of world problems according to homeopathic principles look? What can we learn from our experiences with individuals with regard to solving the current crises? The principles must be the same, because what we apply in homeopathy is only a mirror of the laws according to which the world otherwise functions. So how can we 'treat' a world in crisis? Of course I do not have an answer to this question, but I believe it is our responsibility to start by asking this question: What can be our active role in this process?

One thing is clear: it is not the homeopathic way to fight what we do not want, but to represent what we want to spread and at the same time to reflect the sick condition in the guise of a remedy. It might be a metaphoric remedy, or a conceptual one. It will contain the form and essence of the state we wish to heal. The existence of homeopathy in itself is already a model for what a holistic solution to global problems could look like. And in the medical field it is not just a metaphor, but an actual part of the solution. Along with some of the achievements of modern medicine, homeopathy will have an essential role to play in a future medicine, as will the approaches of other cultures.

154

What practical significance can these considerations have? What can homeopathy mean for the world and in the world?

1: Homeopaths are sitting on a treasure of experience in dealing with crises in a holistic and effective way. In any case, they can testify that every crisis can also be an opportunity and often the best possible chance for change. They could thus become creative and apply their strategies in dealing with crises to political situations and find solutions where none seem visible. They have the knowledge and experience that a problem is only an inverted solution.

2: Since we are usually unable to change the circumstances of our patients' lives – their alienated work, their dysfunctional families, the discriminatory society or a hostile environment – we can at least make them aware of these factors. We can free them from the idea that their disease is their own fault and they just need to make a little more effort to get better or find the better cure or swallow the stronger pill. Seeing reality as it is always makes a first important step towards more health.

3: In order to be credible with this approach, we must also draw our own consequences and arrange our lives differently. I know so many colleagues who work around the clock in their practice and answer an email immediately at two o'clock on Sunday night, who are burnt out, worn to the bone themselves, who take no time for walks, sports, family or creativity because they still 'have to solve cases' – all cases except their own. How credible is it to talk about holistic health under such circumstances?

4: We should see ourselves as part of a large and diverse network and community working to build a different kind of society. As medics we are in a very privileged position and have a large share in the wealth of this society. But we should not let ourselves be seduced by this to believe that we can exercise our 'highest mission' and at the same time benefit from these privileges. Our real place is in the counterculture, in the alternative networks that work, love, fight, heal, discuss, think and write for a healthier planet and a sane, just and human society.

5: To make the system healthy again, homeopathy does not need recognition from an alienated view of the world and medicine. And it also does not help us to let ourselves be put on the defensive, to justify ourselves or our successes in healing or our scientific knowledge. Homeopathy can meet many of the needs of modern and global medicine and fits the way we must think about health, pain, disease and death if humanity is to survive this crisis. We would be well advised to actively disseminate all this and to look for allies wherever we can find them. And this is rather not the case in established orthodox medicine, but in the many groups and networks that also strive for the health of the planet and health.

So what will help us is not to be less homeopathic and to adapt to the common patterns of thinking and become 'complementary' to them, but to become *more* homeopathic in all venues of our lives.

6: Just as our patients are part of a larger whole, so is the art and science of homeopathy part of a larger movement; and it was this from the beginning, if we look at the biography of its founder.[104] Actively participating in this larger movement for alternative and more sustainable lifestyles, business, science and politics makes us part of a vast network of people who need and want our services. As we prepare the ground on which homeopathy can continue to flourish, we also become visible to the many who may need our medical service and would trust us.

7: Doctors, therapists and healers are in a special situation because they have something to give: They help to restore health, relieve pain and release stress. Therefore, our patients will listen to us when we make them aware that our offer can only be a small part of a comprehensive healing process that they must engage with and that the Great Healing can only be a global one. Many people who would otherwise have little interest in the voice of the global community listen us to. Let us use this privilege responsibly.

The future of homeopathy depends on our extending our homeopathic work, our *homoios-pathein*, our compassion, to the whole living world and creating homeopathically what was intended from the very beginning, true healing and health.

Like all other holistic therapy methods rooted in the shamanic or hermetic tradition, homeopathy refers to all aspects that make it a holistic work and a work on the whole, so that "our indwelling, rational mind can freely employ this living, healthy instrument for the higher purpose of our existence". (§9).

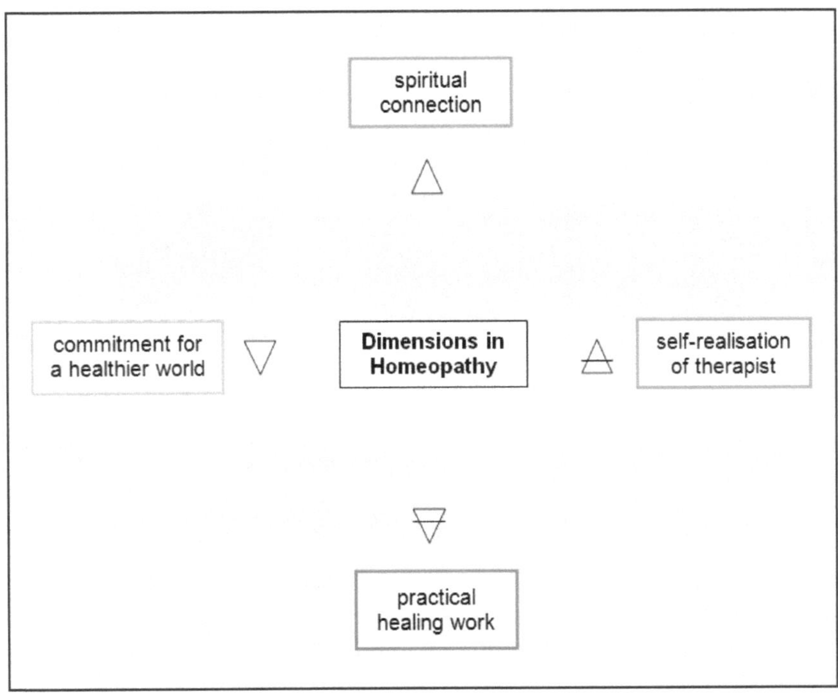

Glossary of Homeopathic Terms

(for more individual terms, contexts and biographies see also
 www.FreeWiki.eu, the encyclopaedia with a holistic perspective)

Acute illness cf. Miasm

Aggravation, (First reaction), cf. chapter 1, section healing process

Allopathy, (for Hahnemann: *Alloeopathie*) is the counter term to homeopathy coined by Hahnemann. However, the term has more polemical than factual value, because it makes little sense to subsume all non-homeopathic healing methods under one word. Allopathy means: healing by the opposite (in contrast to healing with the similar / homeopathy).

Anamnesis (case taking) is the conversation between homeopath and patient to determine all personal details important for the prescription of a remedy. Apart from these, the impression or the atmosphere created during the conversation is certainly just as important. The word *anamnesis* comes from the ancient Greek and means: to bring back from oblivion.

Antidoting means the unintentional suspension or weakening of the action of a homeopathic remedy by certain intolerable other substances (coffee, vinegar); or intentionally by another homeopathic remedy if side effects or proving symptoms of a remedy are to be interrupted (cf. also footnote 74). When homeopathic treatment tries to stimulate the life force, it also depends on what the reaction conditions are like. The reaction possibilities for the healing of a lung disease (to choose a very simple example) are of course more limited in a smoker. Many homeopaths also assume with Hahnemann that a number of foods and stimulants can strongly impair the homeopathic healing possibilities. At the top of this list is coffee, which should be avoided at all costs, but also peppermint and all other essential oils, often vinegar or tea. Probably because Hahnemann smoked himself, tobacco is not one of the substances frowned upon. The handling of these 'antidotes' is differently strict in different homeopaths. Some hardly pay attention to them; others give their patients meticulous rules of conduct. Of course someone who constantly disturbs his energy balance with drugs such as coffee, alcohol or nicotine cannot be healthy in the long run – this insight has nothing to do with homeopathy. But if peppermint tea or any kind of kitchen spices (because Hahnemann also counts them among the antidotes) would make a homeopathic remedy ineffective, then we could not treat most people at all. The experience of many colleagues shows that only rarely and in individual cases is a remedy antidoted by some influence. A well chosen homeopathic remedy works relatively independently from such external events.

Aude sapere was Hahnemann's motto (*Dare to know/to be wise*). Even today there are still some homeopaths who consider Hahnemann's call to dare and be wise of last resort in the literal sense of the word. For them, homeopathic research consists of a text interpretation that is as faithful as possible to Hahnemann's sentence: "Copy it, but copy it exactly". Certainly Hahnemann had such intolerant and dogmatic traits. But the fact that he himself was above all a great reformer and a forward-driving, independent thinker is not reflected in this view of the founder. Such an approach would lead to a sectarian homeopathy, the development of which would be over by the time it began, and which would not do its founder any favours. Therefore, most practitioners follow his motto 'Aude sapere', which is much more suited to his basic attitude and life's work.

Bach flowers, cf. Bach

Bach, Edward (1886-1936) was a British homeopath who had rendered outstanding services to the development of nosodes (cf.). In view of the complexity of finding homeopathic remedies, he then wanted to create a system that would enable even laymen to treat the various ailments and disorders of everyday life in a simple way. He was intuitively led to a total of 38 different medicinal plants, which he prepared into the essences of the *Bach Flower Remedies* by exposing their flowers to sunlight in spring water. The method spread widely in the course of the 20th century and was supplemented by other practitioners with further flowers. Despite some superficial similarities, Bach's new way of healing has little in common with homeopathy. It is based only on personal intuition, not on experience and remedy proving. It is not prescribed on the basis of the rule of similars, but rather allopathically. And the substances are not potentiated.

Boenninghausen, Clemens M.F. von (1785-1864), Hahnemann's pupil, and for whom Hahnemann – apart from his wife Melanie – held the most respect. Boenninghausen developed one of the first repertories and published a number of other writings. Typical for his homeopathic style is to orientate himself predominantly to the modalities and general symptoms.

C -potency, cf. Potentisation

Causa is mentioned in the homeopathic analysis as a clear cause for a sick condition. If, for example, a stone falls on my head, this is considered a causa in the homeopathic sense. However, this only refers to very immediate and easily identifiable effects that lead to a condition which clearly begins with this event. The idea of distinguishing a causa as something special from other backgrounds of a disease is based on the fact that it is the only real *external* effect. A state created by a 'causa' can usually be completely healed with a single remedy.

Chronic disease cf. Miasm

Classical homeopathy. The form of homeopathy, which adheres exactly to the laws and rules of therapy established by Hahnemann, is generally referred to as 'classical'. There is a certain spectrum between the therapists, who rather follow Hahnemann's sentence "Copy it, but copy it exactly", and those who feel more comfortable with his motto "Dare to be wise" (*aude sapere*) and – like Hahnemann himself – continue to research critically and develop the method. In practical terms, 'classically' working homeopaths are usually recognised by the fact that they give only one remedy at a time, that they perform thorough and detailed anamnesis, that they do not mix several methods and that they rely on close observation and listening and not on speculation.

Complex remedies are drugs that are prepared from a mixture of potentiated substances. These are selected on the basis of their reference to certain organs and administered according to orthodox medical criteria, i.e. without taking the simile principle into account. Basically, the so-called complex remedy 'homeopathy' has little in common with Hahnemann's homeopathy.

Constitutional treatment is a very common, but misleading term that does not really arise from homeopathic theory. It usually points to a kind of basic treatment that goes beyond the concrete symptoms. In classical homeopathy, however, existing symptoms are assumed as far as possible. If there are no peculiar, individual symptoms or modalities, but only very general signs of illness, then one can sometimes first only try to prescribe on the basis of the 'constitution' of this person. Of course, there are only a few well-known remedies for which such a clichéd constitution is known (example: Nux vomica is the typical choleric with stress symptoms). In this respect, 'constitutional prescription' in the strict sense is a third choice for lack of good criteria. Many patients even come to the practice with the request: "I am actually healthy, but I would like to know my constitutional remedy". – like my zodiac sign: *Pulsatilla* seeks *Aurum*.

D-potency. Potentisation by dilution in a ratio of 1:10 and shaking (cf. succussion). The D-potencies [in UK: X-potnecies] are a special Central European development of the first half of the 20th century as a concession to scientific thought. "There's more in them." Homeopathically this production is not meaningful and has not become generally accepted. In German pharmacies, especially in complex remedies (cf.), many D-potencies are still used. But with the increasing internationalisation of classical homeopathy, they are slowly disappearing again. In the UK D-potencies are known as X-potencies, again with a dilution ratio of 1:10, and are considered as 'Organ remedies'.

Doctrine of Signatures cf. Theory of Signatures

Dynamis is Hahnemann's expression for the "spiritual life force," as he says. This force has been named in various ways as vital principle, etheric force, Od, Prana, Chi, Ki, animal magnetism. It is the power that permeates all living things and that we have in common with all living beings. Without its action, the physical body decomposes, being subject only to the laws of chemistry.

First reaction, aggravation, cf. chapter 1, section healing process

Follow up is the name for the follow-up appointments after the anamnesis, in which the effect of the given remedy is to be assessed and, if necessary, a second prescription determined.

Globules (also Latin *Globuli*) are the scattered globules of pure sugar, which are usually used as carriers of homeopathic remedies. The last production step of a remedy consists of spraying the desired potency in solution onto such scattered globules. They can be stored well and for a long time and facilitate dosage. The size of these globules varies between the manufacturing companies and is irrelevant for prescription and dosage. The number of globules administered is also unimportant for the healing success. Since it is information and not matter or energy, ten globules are like ten copies of the same poem. If it's valid, one is enough. For psychological and habitual reasons, most practitioners give between three and ten globules.

Hahnemann, Melanie (1800-1878, née Marquise Marie Mélanie d´Hervilly) was Hahnemann's second wife, with whom he ran the practice in Paris during the last ten years of his life. He called her his best student. Unfortunately, as a woman without a medical license, she could only continue practising after his death with great difficulty. Their fate is well described in the book "*A Homeopathic Love Story*" by Rima Handley (cf. Literature).

Hahnemann, Samuel founder of homeopathy. Cf. box in the first chapter.

Hering´s Rule/ Law Frequent observation that a healing process runs from the inside to the outside, from important to less vital organs, from top to bottom and backwards in chronological order is usually referred to as Hering´s Rule or Law. The short-term recurrence of old symptoms is therefore seen as a sign of a desired healing process, as is the shift of symptoms in the directions mentioned above, for example from the lungs to the skin, from the abdomen to the feet.

Hierarchisation is a working technique of homeopathic therapists to bring order to the abundance of symptoms mentioned in the anamnesis.

Isopathy is a healing method of 'like with like' (homeopathy heals with 'similars' not with 'likes'), for example if I would give the nosode *Tuberculinum* for tuberculosis. Vaccination is also an isopathic principle.

Kent, James Tyler (1849 – 1916) can probably be regarded as the most influential homeopath after Hahnemann. He is the author of the most important repertory of homeopathic remedies, the most frequently used series of

162

potencies in the regulation: C 30, C 200, C 1000, C 10,000, and he is still the author of important works on materia medica and homeopathic philosophy. (cf. also box "Historical connections...")

Key symptoms (keynotes) are proven symptoms of a remedy, on which alone the prescription of a remedy is often (but by no means always!) worthwhile.

Life force, s. Dynamis

LM – Potency, cf. Potentisation

Low potency, cf. high potency [pp 32, 88, 90] and Potentisation

Magnetisation means the direct transfer of life force from one person to another. The term, coined by Franz Anton Mesmer (1734-1815), is based on the scientific notion common at the time that there was a close connection or identity between vitality and magnetism. To differentiate between them, animal magnetism was mentioned in part. This connection probably also led Hahnemann to carry out remedy provings with the effect of magnets on the human body. Hahnemann was a convinced advocate of the healing effect of magnetisation and recommended the combination with homeopathic therapy. However, to this day only a few of his students have followed him.

Materia Medica Pura is a list of all individual symptoms obtained in homeopathic remedy trials, without their interpretation or description. In particular, this refers to Hahnemann's own multi-volume work.

Mesmerism, cf. Magnetisation

Miasm, Hahnemann calls the three chronic diseases which he considers to be the 'primal evils' of human suffering: Psora, sycosis, syphilis. Hahnemann's idea was that chronic illness is caused by infection in the body and cannot be cured even by a correct homeopathic acute treatment, i.e. it manifests itself again and again in new symptoms. Most of the occurring ailments are only different manifestations of these three basic chronic diseases, the miasms. An acute illness in the homeopathic sense can only be an illness which is not miasmatically justified, but which occurs as a self-contained unit and can be completely cured with a remedy. A real acute illness either heals on its own and without consequences without any curative measure or leads to death. Almost all acutely occurring health disorders in the usual sense would, however, be classified homeopathically as flare-ups of the basic chronic ailment.

Modalities are the specific circumstances under which a symptom occurs. For the choice of homeopathic remedies it is very important whether a pain always occurs in the morning or in the evening, whether it gets better or worse through heat, etc.

Mother tincture is the initial substance from which the homeopathic remedies are triturated and then succussed, so to speak the potency zero. The term tincture actually refers to an alcoholic solution, but is also used more generally in this context.

Nosodes are homeopathic remedies derived from pathogens. Sterilised and in high potencies these are of course not contagious. The most important nosodes are *Psorinum, Medorrhinum, Syphilinum, Tuberculinum.*

Organon usually refers to Hahnemann's main theoretical work, which in the first edition was called "*Organon of Rational Medicine*" and later "*Organon of the Medical Art*".

Palliation (adj.: palliative) is the term for a medical treatment which, due to an advanced disease condition, no longer has the goal of healing, but only tries to alleviate it.

Placebo (lat.: *I will please*) is the usual term for a fake drug. A placebo effect is defined as the fact that a large proportion of remedies can also be replaced by a substance that is considered medically ineffective, without the effect being diminished. The placebo effect is between 40 and 60 percent for all previously investigated healing methods, both conventional and alternative, depending on the approach of the examination. Interestingly, there is no strong connection between the placebo effect and the suggestibility of the proving subjects, which is usually used as an explanation. – Homeopathy is often accused of only having placebo effect, which has been refuted by a number of studies. (cf. literature on scientific studies and
 www.freewiki.eu/en/index.php?title=Studies_on_homeopathy)

Polychrest (Greek: much used, or also: often healing). In homeopathy, the term polychrest is used to describe those remedies that are constantly used by most practitioners: *Sulphur, Pulsatilla, Calcarea carbonica, Lycopodium, Sepia, Natrum muriaticum* and 30 to 40 others. The so-called small remedies are less well known and are used less frequently. The division has become more and more controversial in recent years and is considered too arbitrary by many homeopaths today.

Potency was first used by Hahnemann as a very general term for all kinds of forces and influences, from the forces of nature, the weather to disease infection, to poison effects and also to remedies. However, in the course of homeopathic history, the term has limited its meaning to remedies which are produced dynamically by means of a precisely defined procedure – cf. potentisation.

Potentisation is the term used by Hahnemann from 1827 for the production of homeopathic remedies. In part, he also spoke of 'dynamising' with the same meaning. Through alternating dilution and rhythmic shaking, the chemical toxic effect of a medicine was reduced on the one hand and its spiritual healing power increased on the other. Potencies are named according to their manufacturing method. If diluted 1:10 per shake, one speaks of a D- [or X-]

164

potency, if diluted 1:100 it is named a C-potency; one dilutes 1:50,000 of a Q- or LM-potency. The D- [or X-] potencies have developed in the camp of homeopathic sceptics who wanted to achieve that more substance is preserved. They do not differ significantly from the C-potencies in their application, but have not become established. The form of preparation used by Hahnemann is that of the C potencies. He only developed the Q-potencies towards the end of his life, because they seemed to be gentler in action to him. These are usually repeated at shorter intervals than the C-potencies and more frequently.

Depending on the school, **high potencies** are called – differently – either those potencies whose degree of dilution is higher than Avogadro's number, i.e. above D24 or C12, or those potencies are meant which are higher than the usual ones, i.e. above C30 and C200.

Cf. also: Succussion.

Psora, cf. Miasma

Q – Potency, cf. Potentisation

Remedy proving cf. section in Chapter 1.

A **Repertory** is a systematic collection of homeopathic symptoms to easily look up which remedies are known to be associated with this symptom. Kent has compiled the most famous repertory. Today there are extended versions. The 'Synthesis' and the 'Complete' are currently the most extensive repertories, which are also available as computer programs.

Return of old symptoms, cf. Hering's Rule/ Law

Schüßler, Wilhelm H. (1821-1898) was a homeopath who tried to simplify homeopathy by low (6X and 12X) potentiated 'biochemical functional agents' which were oriented on cell chemistry. Neither the type of prescription (without simile), nor the notions of illness and health have anything to do with homeopathy.

Succussion is the most important part of making potencies. Hahnemann states that he strongly strikes the vial by hand on a firm but elastic object, such as a leather-bound book. In the meantime, of course, a number of machines have been invented for the innumerable shaking processes that are necessary to produce a C 1000 or even 10,000. Opinions differ as to whether a machine-made potency is just as effective as a hand-shaken one. In any case, the fact is that most homeopathic remedies sold today are produced by machines. In the course of the renaissance of this form of therapy, however, the number of small pharmacies and laboratories all over the world that have set themselves the task of producing homeopathic potencies – and also high potencies – by hand is also growing, as Hahnemann instructed.

Simile/ Similarity principle, rule, cf. 1. chapter

Simillimum refers to the most similar possible remedy for a particular person, whereas Simile simply means one that is similar enough to achieve a satisfactory healing effect. The effect of Simillimum is profound and can change one's whole life. It is undisputed among practitioners that it is very seldom possible to find the true simillimum of a person.

Spagyric is an alchemical method for the production of remedies, which is still used today. As with homeopathic potentisation, this is about freeing the essence of a substance, its essential or spiritual nature from matter.

Suppression in homeopathy means a treatment that causes symptoms to disappear without actually curing the disease. Experience has shown that this leads to a postponement or worsening of the original condition. In principle, any wrong treatment, even a homeopathic one, can have a suppressive effect.

Sycosis, cf. Miasm

Syphilis, cf. Miasm

Theory of signatures is a concept that determines the healing qualities of plants by their outer form, by their juices, colours or other direct properties. Folk medicine has always made use of such analogies. However, the theory of signatures in academic medicine at Hahnemann's time was so degenerated that he spoke out exclusively against it. Many modern homeopaths, on the other hand, use the signatures again, at least as a reminder for complex symptom combinations.

Trituration is the first step in the creation of homeopathic potency. Hahnemann specifies that the first three potentisation steps be carried out by hand grinding the starting material into lactose and then shaking in an alcoholic solution. Only a few manufacturers still comply with this regulation today.

Vithoulkas, Georgos (born 1932) has had a decisive influence on modern homeopathy by emphasising the priority of mood symptoms already established by Hahnemann and by introducing the idea of 'essences' of the individual remedies. Since then, many homeopaths have tried to trace the complex remedy pictures back to clear basic structures or to a basic picture from which most of the symptoms can be derived. For his work in alternative medicine he won the Alternative Nobel Prize.

X-potency, cf. D-potency, cf. Potentisation

Literature

History and Theory of Homeopathy

Apell, Rainer G.: Alchemistische Grillen oder: Die scientifische Erklärung, *wie dieß zugehe.* aus: AHZ Bd.244, 5/1999
id.: Dove Diavolo, Messer Samuel, avete pigliate, tante coglionerie?; Anmerkungen zur Geschichte des Miasmenbegriffs. aus: AHZ Bd.243, 6/1998
id. (Editor): Homöopathie zwischen Heilkunde und Heilkunst, Heidelberg 1997
id. (Editor): Der verwundete Heiler, Heidelberg 1995

Coulter, Harris L.: Hahnemann und die Homöopathie. Eine medizinhistorisch begründete Einführung in die Grundgedanken der homöopathischen Heilkunst, Heidelberg 1994

Dethlefsen, Thorwald: Schicksal als Chance – Das Urwissen zur Vollkommenheit des Menschen, München 1979
Dethlefsen, Thorwald u. Dahlke, Rüdiger: Krankheit als Weg. Deutung und Be-Deutung der Krankheitsbilder, München 1983

Dinges, Martin (Editor): Weltgeschichte der Homöopathie. Länder – Schulen – Heilkundige. München 1996

Eppenich, H.: Samuel Hahnemann und die Beziehung zwischen Homöopathie und Mesmerismus, 1994, ZKH 38, S.153-160

Fritsche, Herbert: Samuel Hahnemann. Idee und Wirklichkeit der Homöopathie, Göttingen 1942/54/79

Gawlik, Willibald: Götter, Zauber und Arznei, Schäftlarn 1994
id.: Samuel Hahnemann. Synchronopse seines Lebens – Geschichte, Kunst, Kultur und Wissenschaft bei Entstehung der Homöopathie 1755-1843, Stuttgart 1996

Gypser, K.-H.: Ein Manuskript Hahnemanns aus seiner Pariser Zeit, 1987, ZKH 31, S.65-73.

Hahnemann, Samuel: Organon, 6. Auflage. (Editor Richard Haehl), Leipzig 1921
id.: Organon of Medicine/ Organon of the Rational Art of Healing
id.: Chronische Krankheiten, Dresden und Leipzig 1835
id.: The Chronic Diseases
id.: Reine Arzneimittellehre, Dresden und Leipzig 1827

Handley, Rima: A Homeopathic Love Story – The Story of Samuel und Mélanie Hahnemann, Berkeley 1990

Kent, James T.: Lectures on Homoeopathic Philosophy, Chicago 1900/ Delhi 1993

Krüger, Andreas/ Achtzehn, Hans-Jürgen: Der homöopathische Ring, Berlin 1997

Lang, Gerhardus: Dynamis und geistartige Heilmittel, in: Homöopathische Einblicke II, 1990, Berlin, ISSN 0937-745X

McCoy, Elmore: JT Kent and the Roots of the Blues, aus: The Homœopath. The Journal of the Society of Homœopaths, No. 68, Winter 1998

Norland, Misha: Open letter to all readers of LINKS concerning the actions of vital energy; in: HomLinks, Vol 13, 3/00, S.138ff.
id.: Symptom as Symbol, Den Haag 1992
id. and Claire Robinson: Signatures, Miasms, Aids: Spiritual Aspects of Homeopathy, Yondercott Press, Gloucestershire 2003
id. and Mani Norland: The Four Elements in Homeopathy: Mappa Mundi of elements and associated temperaments, Yondercott Press, 2007, ISBN 978-0-9544766-2-5

Phatak, S.R.: Materia medica of Homeopathic Medicines, Bombay 1977

Schmidt, J.M.: Homöopathie und Philosophie. in: Scheidewege – Jahresschrift für skeptisches Denken Bd. 20 (1990/91), S. 141-165

Schmitz, Martin (Editor), Strömungen der Homöopathie – Konzepte, Lehrer, Verbreitung, Essen, 2000

Sherr, Jeremy: An Interview with Jeremy Sherr by Nick Churchill, aus: The Homeopath, http://www.thehomoeopath.ndirect.co.uk/articles/jeremy.htm
id.: Dynamics & Methodology of Homoeopathic Provings, Malvern 1994

Van Galen, Emiel: Paracelsus and the Underground Stream in Medical Science, HomLinks 4/95, S.27
id.: Kent´s Hidden Links. The Influence of Emanuel Swedenborg on Homeopathic Philosophy of James Tyler Kent, HomLinks 3/94, S.27

Vithoulkas, Georgos: Homeopathy – Medicine for the new Millennium, 1999, ISBN 978-9608616363
id.: Science of Homeopathy, New York 2000, ISBN 978-0802151209
id.: Essence of Materia Medica: 2nd Edition, New Delhi 2008, ISBN 978-8131902011

Whitmont, Edward C.: Psyche and Substance: Essays on Homeopathy in the Light of Jungian Psychology, Berkeley 1980
id.: Die Alchemie des Heilens, Göttingen 1993

Scientific Research on Homeopathy

„Studies on Homeopathy" – page on www.FreeWiki.eu with extensive literature.

Adams, Peter: Homeopathy - Good Science. How New Science Validates Homeopathy. Gloustershire 2010

Haidvogel, Max: Klinische Forschung in der Homöopathie in den vergangenen 10 Jahren, in: R&D Newsletter der HomInt, Karlsruhe, 2000 – 1/ 2001

Heusser, Peter: Probleme von Studiendesigns mit Randomisierung, Verblindung und Placebogabe. aus: Forschende Komplementärmedizin 1999; 6; 89-102
id.: Kriterien zur Beurteilung des Nutzens von komplementärmedizinischen Massnahmen, zuhanden der Eidg.Leistungskommission des Bundesamtes für Sozialversicherung, 6.Fass. 1998

Ivanovas, Georg: Doppelblind bei alternativen Heilverfahren. in: Deutsches Ärzteblatt 98, Vol. 13 from 30.03.01, pp A-822

Popp, Fritz A.: Biophysikalische Grundlagen der Naturheilkunde, AHZ Bd.245, 4/2000, S. 154

Quinn, Michael: Research on homeopathy and chemistry – Are ice crystals the missing link? HomLinks 3/98

Resch, Gerhard u. Gutmann, Viktor: Wissenschaftliche Grundlagen der Homöopathie, Schäftlarn 1986 (3.Aufl. 1994)

Schiff, Michel: Das Gedächtnis des Wassers – Homöopathie und ein spektakulärer Fall von Wissenschaftszensur, Frankfurt 1997

Shepperd, John: Chaos Theorie: Implication für die Homöopathie, Europäisches Journal für klassische Homöopathie, Nr. 5+6/1996, S.36

Teut, Michael: Homöopathie zwischen Lebenskraft und Selbstorganisation, in: Forschende Komplementärmedizin und Klassische Naturheilkunde Bd.8, Vol. 3, Freiburg 2001, ISSN 1424-7364

Walach, Harald: Homöopathie als Basistherapie. Plädoyer für die wissenschaftliche Ernsthaftigkeit der Homöopathie, Heidelberg 1986

Religious and Intellectual History

Berman, Morris: The Reenchantment of the World, Cornell Univ.Press, London 1981

Duerr, Hans-Peter: Dreamtime: Concerning the Boundary between Wilderness and Civilization. Felicitas Goodman (translator). Oxford and New York (1985) [1978]. Blackwell. ISBN 0-631-13375-5
id.: Traumzeit – Über die Grenze zwischen Wildnis und Zivilisation, Frankfurt 1978
id. (Edit.): Der Wissenschaftler und das Irrationale. Beiträge aus Ethnologie und Anthropologie, Frankfurt 1981, 2 Bände.
id.: Können Hexen fliegen? in: Zeitschrift für Parapsychologie und Grenzgebiete der Psychologie, Jg. 20 Nr. 2, 1978, S.75-91; and in: Unter dem Pflaster liegt der Strand, Bd.3, Berlin, Karin Kramer Verlag, 1976, S.55-82.

Hartmann, Franz: Theophrastus Paracelsus von Hohenheim, Calw o.J.

Kuhn, Thomas S.: The Structure of Scientific Revolutions. Chicago: University of Chicago Press, 1962. ISBN 0-226-45808-3

Mutschler, Hans-Dieter: Physik, Religion, New Age, Würzburg 1992

Pietschmann, Herbert: Das Ende des naturwissenschaftlichen Zeitalters, Stuttgart 1995

Roszak, Theodore: The Voice of the Earth (1992); 2nd edition (2001), Phanes Press, ISBN 978-1890482800

Störig, Hans Joachim: Kleine Weltgeschichte der Wissenschaft, Frankfurt 1982, 2 Bd.

Wichmann, Jörg: Die Renaissance der Esoterik – eine kritische Orientierung, Stuttgart 1990

Whorf, Benjamin Lee: Language, Thought and Reality, Cambridge 1956

Alchemy

Bernus, Alexander von: Alchymie und Heilkunst, Dornach 1994 (Nürnberg 1936)

Biedermann, Hans: Materia Prima – eine Bildersammlung zur Ideengeschichte der Alchemie, Graz 1973

Coudert, Allison: Der Stein der Weisen – Die geheime Kunst der Alchemisten, Bern 1980

Eliade, Mircea: Schmiede und Alchemisten, Stuttgart 1980

id.: Forgerons et Alchimistes, E.Flammarion, Paris (Orig.)

Gebelein, Helmut: Alchemie, München 1991

Jung, Carl Gustav: Psychologie und Alchemie, Olten 1975

Priesner, Carl u. Figala, Karin: Alchemie – Lexikon einer hermetischen Wissenschaft, München 1998

Scherer, Richard (Editor), Alchymia, alchemistische Texte des 16. und 17. Jahrhunderts, Mössingen 1988

Schütt, Hans-Werner: Auf der Suche nach dem Stein der Weisen, München 2000

Tomberg, Valentin: Die großen Arcana des Tarot. Meditationen, Freiburg 1983

Shamanism

Bates, Brian: Wyrd – Der Weg eines angelsächsischen Zauberers, München 1984
id.: The Wisdom of the Wyrd, Rider, 1996

Biedermann, Hans: Hexen – Auf den Spuren eines Phänomens, Graz 1974

Castaneda, Carlos: The Teachings of Don Juan: A Yaqui Way Of Knowledge, 1968
id.: A Separate Reality, Further Conversations with Don Juan
id.: Journey to Ixtlan, Simon & Schuster, New York 1972

Eliade, Mircea: Schamanismus und archaische Ekstasetechnik, Frankfurt 1975
id.: Shamanism: Archaic Techniques of Ecstasy, Princeton University Press, Princeton, 2004
Orig.: Le chamanisme et les techniques archaïques de l'extase, Paris 1951

Ginzburg, Carlos: Die Benandanti – Feldkulte und Hexenwesen im 16. und 17.Jahrhundert, Frankfurt 1980

Golowin, Sergius: Die Weisen Frauen – die Hexen und ihr Heilwissen, München 1982

Kaiser, Rudolf: Indianische Heilkunst – Pflanzen, Rituale und Heilungsbilder nordamerikanischer Schamanen, Freiburg 1996

Kharitidi, Olga: Das weiße Land der Seele, München 1996

Müller, Indianische Welterfahrung, Frankfurt 1981

Schamanische Wege der Heilung – Hexen, Druiden, weise Frauen. Connection special Nr. 56, V/01.

Schwarzer Hirsch: The Sacred Pipe, 1956

Tedlock, Dennis & Barbara: Teachings from the American Earth: Indian Religion and Philosophy. New York 1975, Liveright/Norton

Wisselinck, Erika: Hexen – warum wir so wenig von ihrer Geschichte erfahren und was davon auch noch falsch ist, München 1986

History and Sociology of Medicine and Health Care Law

Biedermann, Hans: Medicina magica – Metaphysische Heilmethoden in spätantiken und mittelalterlichen Handschriften, Graz 1972

Ehrenreich, Barbara & English, Deidre: Witches, Midwives, and Nurses: A History of Women Healers, 1972, ISBN 978-1558616615

Eckart, Wolfgang U.: Geschichte der Medizin, Berlin Heidelberg 1990

Goldammer, Kurt: Paracelsus in der deutschen Romantik, Wien 1980

Groddeck, Georg: Verdrängen und heilen. Aufsätze zur Psychoanalyse und zur psychosomatischen Medizin, Frankfurt 1988

Illich, Ivan: Medical Nemesis. 1975. ISBN 0-394-71245-5

Ivanovas, Georg: „Contributions of System-Theory to the Understanding of Therapy and Health", Dissertation, unpublished

Jütte, Robert: Geschichte der alternativen Medizin – Von der Volksmedizin zu den unkonventionellen Therapien von heute, München 1996

Nager, Frank: Der heilkundige Dichter – Goethe und die Medizin, Zürich München 1990

Piechowiak, Helmut: Ethische Probleme der modernen Medizin, Mainz 1985

Rösch, Bruno: Die Stellung der Erfahrungsheilkunde aus verfassungs- und verwaltungsrechtlicher Sicht. Dargestellt am Beispiel der geistig Heilenden, Basel und Frankfurt 1994

Abbreviations of periodicals
AHZ = Allgemeine Homöopathische Zeitung. Wissenschaftliche und praktische Homöopathie. ISSN 0175-7881, K.F.Haug Verlag, Heidelberg.
ZKH = Zeitschrift für Klassische Homöopathie. Grundlagen, Materia medica, Praxis. ISSN 0935-0853, K.F.Haug Verlag, Heidelberg.
HomLinks = Homœopathic Links. International Journal for Classical Homeopathy, ISSN 1019-2050

Publications by Jörg Wichmann

"Homeopathy and the World"
You find texts and considerations on up-to-date issues in my Blog on-line: **www.provings.info/blog1_en/**

"FreeWiki"
The encyclopaedic portal **www.FreeWiki.eu/en/** presents homeopathic and holistic facts and terms in a correct and neutral way that have been manipulated in Wikipedia.

Articles by the author on homeopathic topics having been published in different homeopathic journals (like Homeopathic Links, Spectrum of Homeopathy) see: **www.provings.info/en/buecher.html**

Footnotes

1 The corresponding WHO study is available at:
 http://apps.who.int/iris/bitstream/handle/10665/43108/9241562862_map.pdf.
2 In this book, homeopathy is only understood as the so-called "classical" homeopathy founded by Hahnemann more than two hundred years ago. Many other curative methods, such as isopathy, complex remedy "homeopathy", naturopathy in general, organotropic low potency homeopathy based on materialistic science or other curative methods based on potentiated remedies, have gone other ways and are neither treated nor evaluated in this book.
3 On the meaning of dynamis at Hahnemann see in detail: Lang, G., *Dynamis und geistartige Heilmittel.*
4 All of these remedies are now being collected in one large online database www.provings.info.
5 Detailed and excellent instructions for correct drug proving according to Hahnemann´s criteria can be found in Sherr, J.: *Dynamics & Methodology.*
6 In the meantime, the website www.provings.info has collected an almost complete collection of all drug provings since Hahnemann and made them accessible either as a direct link or as a reference. As of summer 2019 there are more than 6000 entries for more than 2400 proved remedies.
7 cited after Gebelein, *Alchemie*, p.216
8 Dethlefsen /Dahlke – *Krankheit als Weg*, p. 85f
9 "In the healthy state of man, the spiritual life force (autocracy), which as dynamis invigorates the material body (organism), prevails unrestrictedly and keeps all its parts in admirably harmonious course of life, in feelings and activities, so that our inherent, rational spirit can freely use this living, healthy instrument for the higher purpose of our existence." (Organon §9)
10 Augustine, *Confessions* XI / 14
11 Susanne Diez, Jörg Wichmann: *Im Zentrum Lebenskraft*. Zwei Studien zu Theorie und Praxis, Teil A. Documenta Homoeopathica Band 30, 2014, S. 1 ff, Wien 2014, ISBN 978-3-99002-002-9
12   Under <www.homoeopathie-konkret.de/Resources/Wissenschaft-3.08.pdf> and printed in *Abschied von der Lebenskraft*, Homöopathie Konkret 3/08; 97-102
13 This chapter is a revised version of part B of an article: Susanne Diez, Jörg Wichmann: *Im Zentrum Lebenskraft*. Zwei Studien zu Theorie und Praxis, Teil A. Documenta Homoeopathica Band 30, 2014, S. 1 ff, Wien 2014, ISBN 978-3-99002-002-9
14 Vijnana is how Buddhists refer to ‚life force' which they equate with consciousness. Prana, in yoga or Indian medicine, is the source of energy for the body. In T'ai Chi the lower tantien is the energy centre of the body (and is situated where Hahnemann indicates – between navel and pubes). Hahnemann was in the right area – the Hara.

15 Chi has a certain intensity, which can be measured, for example, in pulse diagnosis. But Chi also has structural aspects such as the characteristics of the five elements and the flow in the body differentiated by the meridians.
In the Indian system of yoga, in which the life force is called prana, we find the differentiation into chakras and nadis.
16 Bio-energetic therapies according to the teachings of Wilhelm Reich.
17 For the essence of the life force called orgone energy see the websites of the Wilhelm Reich Institute Vienna <www.wilhelmreich.at/wilhelm-reich/lebensenergie> and of Vittorio Nicola <www.w-reich.de> as well as the works of Wilhelm Reich himself. As a book: Bernd Senf, Die Wiederentdeckung des Lebendigen: Erforschung der Lebensenergie durch Reich, Schauberger; Lakhovsky et.al., Aachen 2003. However, many internet pages on the subject are very obscure and not particularly suitable for an objective occupation with the subject of life energy.
18 Cf. the page on "Studies on homeopathy" in www.FreeWiki.eu/en/.
19 Such pseudoscientific attempts to explain the homeopathic mechanisms of action can unfortunately be found in many homeopathy books. Well-intentioned, however, they are predominantly based on a lack of knowledge of scientific theory. Neither has modern physics refuted the materialistic view of the world, as is often claimed (how should it?), nor can pseudoscientific concepts such as "energies" or "molecular resonances" (cf. Vithoulkas, *Medizin der Zukunft*) hide the fact that there are few serious approaches to the materialistic understanding of homeopathy. - The justification of these connections would go beyond the scope of this book and should be given elsewhere. See also the chapter: Materialistic Science and Homeopathy.
On the pseudoscience of "New Age" physics, see Mutschler, *Physik.*
20 The topic is discussed in more detail and in the integration into other traditions in Wichmann, *Renaissance der Esoterik.*
21 For the condensation of the world views into the language see: Whorf: *Language, Thought and Reality*; and Tedlock: *Teachings from the American Earth.*
22 Eliade, *Schmiede und Alchemisten*
For example, Eliade says: "We believe that the ideas concerning the earth mother and the ores and metals, but above all the *experience of* the archaic man who worked in the mine, in the furnace and in the blacksmith's shop, are to be regarded as one of the main sources of alchemy ... But they were also mysteries, because on the one hand they embraced the holiness of the cosmos and on the other hand they were passed on through initiations as 'professional secrets' ". (p. 149f)
23 cf. for example the very old legends around Wayland the Smith
24 cf. *Alchymia*, p. 17
25 cf. Jung and Eliade
26 C.G. Jung, *Psychologie und Alchemie*, Olten 1975, Orig.: 1944, Ges.Werke Vol. 12
27 Eliade, *Schmiede*, p. 150
28 for example Alexander von Bernus, see also in: Gebelein, *Alchemie*
29 cf. for example the first issues of the magazine *Quinta Essentia*, 1984, or the books of Fra Albertus.

30 Good examples can be found in Jung, *Alchemie*, and in Biedermann, *Materia Prima – eine Bildersammlung zur Ideengeschichte der Alchemie*, Graz 1973

31 cf. v.Bernus' sharp criticism of Jung's spiritualising interpretation of alchemy: "In contrast to Jung's erroneous and, seen from a higher spiritual point of view, completely superficial assertion that the alchymistic instructions and imaging are exclusively about interpretations of mental development processes, one who is familiar with the alchymistic contexts of experience and has followed the alchymistic path of experience also in the sense of practical alchemy and who has not only theorised about its sign language and symbolic world, states: The so-called Philosopher's Stone, the mysterious elixir, is producible." (Bernus, p.49)
"However, by denying the realisation of the alchemistic aspiration within the material world, because he has not experienced it himself, he – this is the accusation made against him – goes against the law of correspondences: as above, so below." (Bernus, p. 51)

32 Gebelein, *Alchemie*, p.56

33 The text is late antique with probably much older roots. One suspects partly Arabic sources (cf.: *Die großen Arkana des Tarot*, p.23f), and it is traced back by legend up to Apollonius of Thyana. The Latin version can be found in: *Alchymia*. – Further explanations also in Wichmann, *Esoterik*. The English translation here mainly follows the translation of Isaac Newton of his *Alchemical Papers* as to be found in the King's College Library Cambridge Univ., cited in Wikipedia, with some minor changes.

34 An excellent modern representation of the esoteric basic laws can be found in Dethlefsen, *Schicksal als Chance*.

35 Krüger/Achtzehn: *Der homöopathische Ring*, p.36

36 cf. in detail Dethlefsen, *Schicksal*, and Wichmann, *Esoterik*

37 Heiner Hastedt: *Das Leib-Seele-Problem*, in: Appell, *Der verwundete Heiler*, p. 124ff and see the later chapter on the modern Idealism of Bernardo Kastrup *"The End of the Mechanistic World view"*

38 I use the term "real" here according to C.G.Jung: "Real is what works."

39 This connection is laid out in great detail in Appell, *Alchemistische Grillen*, *AHZ* 5/1999.

40 Appell (e.g. in *Homöopathie zwischen Heilkunde und Heilkunst*) rightly speaks of the scientistic self-misunderstanding of homoeopathy.

41 C.G. Jung was faced with the same problem within psychology. He solved it a lot like Hahnemann. With the help of his conceptually newly introduced 'archetypes', he came back to the concept of the ancient deities (or planets, if you look at it astrologically/alchemistically) and reinstated them as the rulers of the deeper soul layers. And with the help of his construction of 'synchronicity', he gave them access to external reality. One can assume, however, that Jung was more aware of this trick than Hahnemann, who seems to have actually suppressed his alchemical roots. Accordingly, it took longer within homeopathy until the connections became transparent.

42 cf. for example in Tischner, *Geschichte*, or in Appell, *Alchemistische Grillen*

43 Neagu, Michael: *Von der Ethnohomöopathie zur postkommunistischen Vielfalt: Rumänien.* in: Dinges (Ed.) – *Weltgeschichte der Homöopathie*, S. 259

44 cf. in greater detail in Kent, *Lectures*, S. 69ff

45 The bearers of practical healing knowledge had been almost completely exterminated in Europe up to Hahnemann's time in the course of the systematic persecutions of witches. Paracelsus still did have the opportunity to experience them and he said that he had all his medical knowledge from the Wise Women. Hahnemann could no longer get to know them, and the writings of Paracelsus were written in a language that was hardly comprehensible to a child of the Enlightenment. The medical studies at Hahnemann's time were purely theoretical, and the sick were treated on the basis of the old texts by Galen and others, which of course were also based on remnants of the old healing knowledge, but had lost the connection to practical experience and could therefore easily be misinterpreted, for example when the pictorial language of the theory of signatures was taken literally.

46 Whitmont, *Psyche*, p. 56f

47 "Spiritual Forces/Cosmic Energies: Those who believe in it will not find it difficult to accept homeopathy. Personally, I cannot believe it, and as a Christian I must even reject this other faith.

Alternative medicine and Christianity: For Christians even more crucial questions arise than indicated in the evaluation: Yin and Yang, the principle behind many ideological methods (e.g. acupuncture) are gods in China. Who is behind cosmic energies? Can a Christian really accept another faith as the basis of therapy? Here are two statements that apply specifically to Christians: Nowhere in the Bible is there a neutral area. Either someone belongs in the kingdom of God or in the kingdom of darkness. There's no quasi-neutral ground to move on. The same applies to forces and energies. There are only two methods of healing in the Bible: On the one hand, scientific medicine in the sense: Take a medicine that will help you (e.g. the fig cake with Hezekiah (2 Kings 20:8) or the wine that Paul recommends Timothy for his weak stomach (1 Timothy 5:23)). On the other hand, supernatural healing through faith, laying on of hands, mixing a saliva mash, forgiveness of sins, banning, exorcism of demons... These supernatural healings are never related to energies, but as unusual as they are in individual cases, they always occur directly in connection with God as the doer."
Expressed by an unauthorised Christian on the Internet:
<http://home.t-online.de/home/Schulz.1/zvd.htm?zdc.htm>
Dr. Jörg Dechert comments more moderately in
 <http://www.nikodemus.net/article.php?article=29&result=37927&page=1>
"On the one hand, homeopathy brings a legitimate concern into medicine which also accommodates the biblical image of man – this is the close interweaving of body, soul and spirit which is often considered dissolved by "conventional medicine" in its scientific tradition. The sometimes expressed accusation of "unscientificness" does not disqualify homoeopathy from a Christian point of view – for also many biblical truths are criticised as unscientific. On the other hand, some proponents of homeopathy simultaneously represent a more or less esoteric world view. We are talking about "self-healing powers" or "harmony with the energy of nature", and it is not always easy to decide when the border to an unbiblical spirituality is crossed here. So – as so often in life as a Christian – you will have to examine in individual cases (this is also a part of

"being sent into the world") which concrete spiritual attitudes "stand behind" homeopathy. But even if someone openly represents esoteric ideas under the outward appearance of homeopathy, God's word is valid, namely that... "...neither death nor life, neither angels nor principalities nor powers, neither the present nor the future, neither the high nor the low nor any other creature can separate us from the love of God which is in Christ Jesus our Lord." (Romans 8, 38+39)."
What seems strange here is that self-healing powers and harmony with nature per se are already classified as unchristian.
48 Hahnemann in "Äskulap auf der Waagschale", and see also Organon §9.
49 Gebelein, *Alchemie*, p.374f
50 Bernus, p. 69
51 A good example of this is the "*Marburg Declaration*" against Homeopathy, with which not only a whole committee of academically active physicians made themselves ridiculous in public by their almost incomprehensible ignorance in questions of scientific theory, but which also shows the still existing connection between the formation of myths and power.
Declaration of the Marburg Medical Faculty against Homeopathy from 1992 "Homeopathy as heresy and deception of the patient."
"The Department of Human Medicine of the Philipps-University Marburg rejects "homeopathy" as a heresy. Only as such can it be the subject of teaching. In this sense, the range of courses offered in Marburg is sufficient. However, we see the danger that "neutrality" and "balance" will be demanded of us in this field, and we are not prepared to abandon our position of logical thinking in favour of unreasonableness.
We do not regard homeopathy as an unconventional method that requires further scientific examination. We proved it, homeopathy has nothing to do with naturopathy. It is often claimed that homeopathy is based on a "different way of thinking". This may be so. However, the rational foundation of homeopathy consists of errors (rule of similarity, drug picture, potentisation by dilution). Their concept is to pass these errors off as truth. Its active principle is the deception of the patient, reinforced by the self-deception of the practitioner.
We do not deny that "homeopathy" can sometimes achieve therapeutic effects, which are so-called placebo effects. Now one might object: What do we care about the principle of action and the rational foundation, when the only thing that matters is the effect? According to this logic, our medical students should also be taught and proved in the following subjects: Chirology (significance of the palm lines for personality structure and holistic medicine); iris diagnostics; reincarnation therapy; astrological health counselling (significance of the zodiac signs for the tendency to certain diseases). With all these methods, whose principle of action is deception, not only therapeutic effects can be achieved, but also considerable sales. These methods are just as incompatible with the spiritual foundations of the Philipps-Universität Marburg as "homeopathy" is.
We do not claim that the science we represent can explore and explain everything, but it does enable us to explain that homeopathy cannot explain anything. A superstition the general public has been talked into believing by interested parties may see this

178

differently and wish for balance and cooperation between "homeopathy" and "allopathy". The guiding principle of our actions, however, is not a superstition that lives in the population and is fueled by journalism, but human reason, which tells us that the words "homeopathy" and "allopathy" do not denote a contradiction, but a conceptual world without a real basis. We would like to point out that Philipps-Universität Marburg does not teach "allopathy" either.
If our university could be forced to offer the subject of "homeopathy" in a neutral sense, it would betray its mission and destroy its rational foundation. A neutral education in "homeopathy" therefore does not take place and is also not enforceable."
(Excerpt from the Internet
<http://oehwww.uibk.ac.at/natwi/pharm/bunsi/0195/marburg.htm or: http://www.mh-hannover.de/student-alt/homoeo/marburg.html> and from Robert Jütte, Wege der Alternativen Medizin, p.164ff.)
52 This supposed longevity is currently (2019) being challenged and it remains yet unclear whether differentiated clusters of water molecules can stay for nano seconds only of for years.
53 A detailed bibliography of such studies, metastudies and discussions can be found in the page "Studies on Homeopathy" in www.FreeWiki.eu.
54 cf. the detailed work of G. Ivanovas on this topic
55 Schuck, Dipl.-Psych. Dr. med. Dr. phil. Peter; Müller, Dipl.-Psych. Dr. phil. Horst; Resch, Prof. Dr. med. habil. Karl-Ludwig: *Wirksamkeitsprüfung: „Doppelblindstudien" und komplexe Therapien,* in: *Deutsches Ärzteblatt* 98, Heft 30 vom 27.07.01, pp.A-1942.
56 cf. also the different works of H.Walach on this issue
57 cf. the articles on „Double-blind studies" and „Replication crisis" on www.FreeWiki.eu.
58 cf. https://www.homoeopathie-online.info/schweiz-homoeopathie-ist-wirksam-zweckmaessig-und-wirtschaftlich/
59 cf. also the detailed page "Studies on homeopathy" in www.FreeWiki.eu
60 Interestingly, Hahnemann had already developed the idea of microorganisms that were involved in the disease process long before they could actually be detected. Hahnemann was, by the way, a well-known chemist and pharmacist and scientifically at the height of his time in every respect – which he also attached great importance to. But despite such forward-looking ideas as the idea of microorganisms as pathogens, it remained clear to Hahnemann that the nature of the disease itself was immaterial. He stressed that unceasingly.
61 from the spiritual comic "*Die sieben Wurzeln Cerric McKardacs*" by Fred Hageneder, Verlag Neue Erde, Rotenbergstr. 33, D-66111 Saarbrücken.
62 In the Marburg Declaration already quoted, doctors actually describe homeopathy as a "heresy" and thus take up the religious language of the Inquisition.
63 cf. also Appell, R.: *Homöopathie und psychoanalytische Initiation – zwischen Selbsterkenntnis und Selbstüberhebung.* In: Appell, *Der verwundete Heiler*
64 cf. Eliade, *Schamanismus*, p. 14. This book by Eliade has been the standard work on shamanism for decades and has shaped the modern use of terms.

65 "When the soul kidnapped by ghosts or the dead has to be found again, the shaman leaves his body and goes to the underworld or to the area where the kidnapper lives. (...) so that the shaman can catch the sick man's soul and bring it back to the body." Eliade, *Schamanismus*, p. 314

66 Eliade, *Schamanismus*, p.52

67 Compare for example the books and the "shamanic" music of the American "city shaman" Gabrielle Roth, or the booklet *"Schamanische Wege der Heilung"* of the magazine *Connection*.

68 This applies, by the way, regardless of whether these works are genuine or fictional: the experiences described in them as such are genuine and are often confirmed in other literature. But nowhere else are they so compactly and comprehensibly (and excitingly) brought together as with Castaneda. In this respect his first books are worthwhile, whether one believes him or not: Ethnologically they are good.

69 Eliade, *Schamanismus*, p. 96

70 Eliade, *Schamanismus*, p. 98, 113

71 Phatak, S.R.: *Materia medica*, S.vii

72 Eliade, *Schamanismus*, p. 288

73 with Nick Churchill in: *The Homeopath*

74 The list of substances to be avoided at Hahnemann, for example, also contains most kitchen spices and many other things that hardly any homeopath pays attention to today. And the experiences collected in the Materiae medicae describe many specifics for individual remedies, which are also usually not taken into account − among these, for example, vinegar is a very frequently observed antidote, which I have never heard of being banned. Instead, coffee and mint are generally banned, which clearly shows that ritual concepts of purity rather than empirical criteria are followed here. − In saying this, I am not saying that the taboos are unimportant or ineffective; on the contrary. I only consider it important to be clear about the structures of one's own work, especially if one wants to discuss meaningfully with representatives of other disciplines.

To make clear how far Hahnemann goes in his prohibitions, here is his list from Organon §260: "Coffee, fine Chinese and other herbal teas; beers made with plant substances inappropriate for the condition of the sick person, so-called fine liqueurs prepared with medicinal spices, all kinds of punch, spiced chocolate, fragrant water and perfumeries of some kind, strongly scented flowers in the room, tooth powder composed of medicines and tooth alcohol. Odoriferous cushions, highly spiced dishes and sauces, spiced baked cookies and frozen foods with medicinal substances, e.g. coffee, vanilla, etc. prepared, raw, medicinal herbs on soups, vegetables of herbs, roots and sprouting stems (such as asparagus with long, green tips), hop sprouts and all vegetables possessing medicinal power, celery, parsley, sorrel, dragon, all kinds of onions, etc. Old cheeses and animal foods which are in decay (meat and fat from pigs, ducks and geese, or overly young veal and sour foods; salads of all kinds), which have medicinal side effects, are just as much to be removed from sick people of this kind as any excess, even that of sugar and table salt, as spiritual drinks which are not diluted with much water. Heated rooms, sheep wool clothing on the skin, a sedentary way of life in the locked-up room air, or more often, just passive movement (by riding, driving, swinging), excessive child suckling, long nap in the lying position (in beds), reading in a horizontal position, nightlife, uncleanness, unnatural lust, exasperation by reading slippery writings, onanism or, be it out of superstition, be it to prevent the generation of children in marriage, imperfect or completely suppressed sexual intercourse; objects of anger, grief, annoyance, passionate gambling, exaggerated effort of mind and body, immediately after the meal; swampy residential area and dull rooms; meagre starving and so on. All these things must be avoided or removed if healing is not to be hindered or made impossible. Some of my imitators seem to make the patient's diet unnecessarily difficult by forbidding even more, rather indifferent things, which is not to be condoned."

75 For such handling of the remedies and remote effects see also the dispute in Norland, M.: *Open letter...*

76 Krüger/ Achtzehn: *Der homöopathische Ring*, p.35

77 Jeremy Sherr, *Neon*, ISBN: 9781908127075, p.6

78 We must bear in mind that the concept of "gravity" only describes and does not explain the regular falling down of things, just as the concept of sychronicity or analogy does with the meaningful chains of events. We have become so accustomed to many concepts of the scientific theory system that we regard them as explanations, although they are only terms for regular observations. We can even give a mathematical regularity of gravity, but that doesn't explain anything.

79 Eppenich, p. 153-54

80 Schmitz, M., *Strömungen*, p.17

81 Hahnemann, in: Gypser, p.72

82 Hahnemann, in: Gypser, p.72

83 Krüger/ Achtzehn: *Der Homöopathische Ring*, p.35

84 Roszak, *The Voice of the Earth*, p.64

85 Rösch, p.36

86 The first three volumes of Castaneda are an eloquent example and once again recommended for the accompanying inner struggles. Or the travelogues of Alexandra David-Neel.

87 See the fascinating considerations Pirsig makes about the cultural immune system in the novel Lila. Pirsig, Robert M.: Lila: *An Inquiry into Morals*, 1991, p. 62ff

88 A famous saying of king Frederick the Great of Prussia when he installed free choice and tolerance of religions: "Es solle jeder nach seiner Façon selig werden".

89 www.impfschaden.info/krankheiten-impfungen/hepatitis-b/impfung.html

90 www.freewiki.eu/en/index.php?title=Sceptical_movement

91 www.csicop.org/specialarticles/show/the_skepkon_report_with_susan_gerbic#footer

92 www.skepkon.org/programm

93 www.csicop.org/specialarticles/archive/category/guerrilla_scepticism

94 www.sceptic.com/get_involved/fix_wikipedia/

95 www.csicop.org/specialarticles/show/the_skepkon_report_with_susan_gerbic#footer

96 A book for those who can read German, in which these thoughts are deepened in partly quite an amusing way, is: "*Angst vor Globuli?*" by HaJo Fritschi, Books on Demand and Kindle, 2017. ISBN 978-3-7431-3508-6.

97 Together with my Canadian colleague Iain Marss and my Indian colleague Manish Bhatia, I commented on this in detail in "*The Sacred Cows of Homeopathy*" in *HomeopathicLinks* Winter 2012, www.homoeopathie-wichmann.de/Artikel/Sacred%20Cows%20Article.pdf.

98 Re Bernardo Kastrup and his articles and books see the article on Bernardo Kastrup in www.FreeWiki.eu/en and www.bernardokastrup.com/

99 cf. http://isharonline.org/hard-problem

100 cf. for example, the efforts to establish criteria for "complementary medicine" in Switzerland: Rösch, *Die Stellung der Erfahrungsheilkunde*, and Heusser, *Kriterien zur Beurteilung*.

101 cf. also the fascinating work of W. Müller: *Indianische Welterfahrung*.

To elucidate my point, I would like to quote a longer extract from Whorf (*Language, Thought and Reality*, p.18), which comes to a similar assessment from a linguistic point of view:

"One significant contribution to science from the linguistic point of view may be the greater development of our sense of perspective. We shall no longer be able to see a few recent dialects of the Indo-European family, and the rationalizing techniques elaborated from their patterns, as the apex of the evolution of the human mind, nor their present wide spread as due to any survival from fitness or to anything but a few events of history – events that could be called fortunate only from the parochial point of view of the favored parties. They, and our own thought processes with them, can no longer be envisioned as spanning the gamut of reason and knowledge but only as one constellation in a galactic expanse. A fair realization of the incredible degree of diversity of linguistic system that ranges over the globe leaves one with an inescapable feeling that the human spirit is inconceivably old; that the few thousand years of history covered by our written records are no more than the thickness of a pencil mark on the scale that measures our past experience on this planet; that the events of these recent millenniums spell nothing in any evolutionary wise, that the race has taken no sudden spurt, achieved no commanding synthesis during recent millenniums, but has only played a little with a few of the linguistic formulations and views of nature bequeathed from an inexpressibly longer past. Yet neither this feeling nor the sense of precarious dependence of all we know upon linguistic tools which themselves are largely unknown need be discouraging to science but should, rather, foster that humility which accompanies the true scientific spirit, and thus forbid that arrogance of the mind which hinders real scientific curiosity and detachment."

102 This chapter has been published in a similar form in issue 1/2018 of *Homoeopathic Links*.

103 Hahnemann uses the term "höchster Beruf", which would better be translated as "highest profession", but as in the German "Beruf" we also hear "Berufung" with the root word "Ruf", the deeper meaning of which is: "our highest call[ing]" in the sense of being called to something or being set on a quest, so here it comes near to the above translation of "mission". (*Organon* §1, as translated by Dudgeon in Hahnemann, Samuel. *Organon*, 5th Ed., Headland: London 1849)

104 Hahnemann was not only a doctor, but was also involved in many areas of society. He was a Freemason, where in his time the most important intersection of Enlightenment philosophy and hermetic spirituality lay. He tried to develop new and creative and above all more humane methods of treatment for mentally confused people, which was groundbreaking for his epoch. He repeatedly risked his reputation and economic existence to stand up for what he saw as the truth and as his rights, e.g. to produce remedies himself. In addition to homeopathic remedies, he also worked with mesmerism, which in his time was considered a new and progressive but controversial method.

Acknowledgement

Although this book was written by one author, it is – like most works –
a collaborative work in its depth. It was born as the fruit of countless
conversations and encounters and grew with life in our practice and
conversations in working groups and seminars. I thank my friend Georg
for many suggestions, corrections and the critical review of the
manuscript.
In particular, I thank my wife, best friend, colleague and critic
Angelika: without our long journey together in homeopathy, this book
would be unthinkable. I wouldn't have started it without your
encouragement. You kept the practice going so I could write it. Your
way of working has always been a model of healing for me. And your
rigorous editing has made the text easy and fluid.
And I would like to thank all our patients who have given us a
trustworthy insight into their life history and their suffering, enabling us
to trace the connections described here.

For the English edition I thank my friend and colleague Jenni Tree, who
has not only improved the language a lot, but also improved and
sharpened my thoughts with her vast knowledge of homeopathy and her
philosophical understanding.

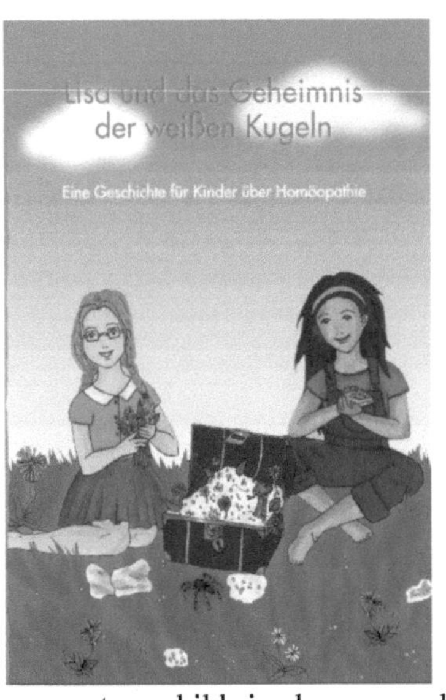

Lisa and the Mystery of the Little White Globules

- A Story about Homeopathy for Children

Narrated by Jörg Wichmann

Illustrations by Melina Meyer

Although this book is a children's book, it is not intended exclusively for children. An explanatory image, an example that makes sense to a child, is also more plausible for a deeper understanding of adults than a theory. We have only really understood those things that we can explain in very simple terms. Trust does not arise in the mind, but at least needs a plausible basis there. And such a basis must also be reasonable for a child.

If homeopathy in general is to be taken seriously and accepted, then we also need the child's imagination, which determines our fears, desires and decisions deep within us all. The aim of this book is to contribute to this. It will also be interesting for many adults who read it aloud for a child or read it along.

Narayana Publishing House, Blumenplatz 2, D-79400 Kandern, Germany

ISBN 978-3-941706-84-2

published in German, English, Dutch, Persian